HASHIMOTO'S DIET COOKBOOK

FOR THE NEWLY DIAGNOSED

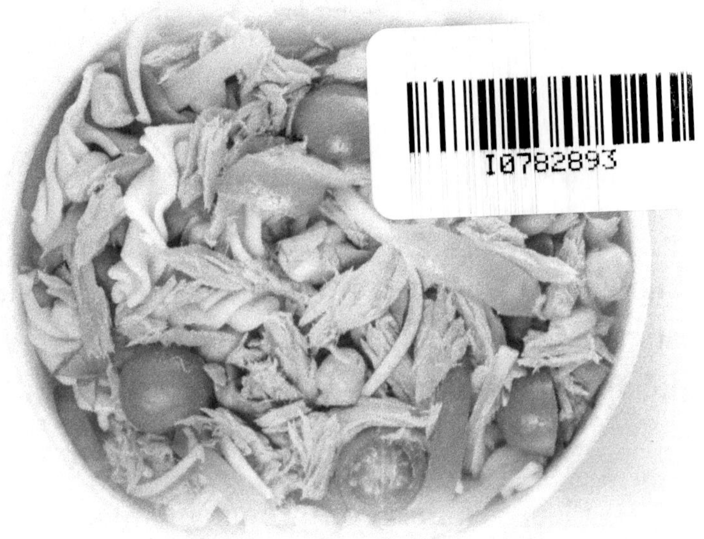

The Latest Powerful Recipes For Thyroid Healing And Eliminate Toxins With Healthy Meals To Boost The Immune System

KEVIN S. MAXWELL

EMAIL ME!

I know that exploring topics that involve food and nutrition can often lead to questions and uncertainty. I invite you to contact me with any questions you may have. I'm here to assist.

Please contact me through email at **kevinmaxwelldiet@gmail.com**, and I will try my best to respond to you within 24 hours.

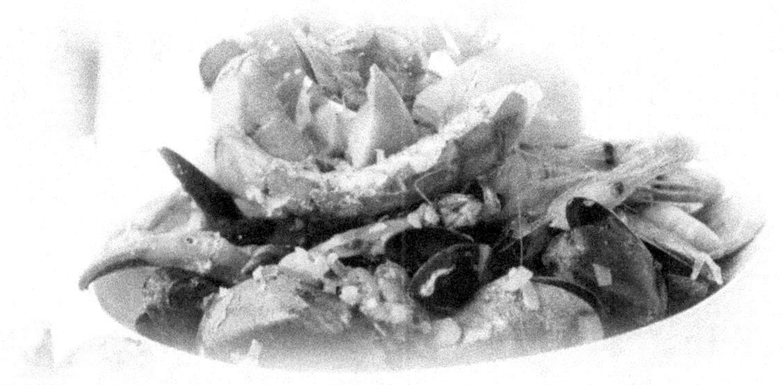

HOW TO USE THIS COOKBOOK?

Familiarize Yourself: Begin by familiarizing yourself with the introductory sections of the cookbook. This may include understanding the basics of Hashimoto's disease, its impact on thyroid health, and the role of nutrition in managing symptoms.

Browse Recipes: Take a leisurely browse through the cookbook's recipe sections. Each recipe is categorized for easy navigation, such as breakfast, lunch, dinner, snacks, and desserts. Pay attention to any special icons or labels denoting gluten-free, dairy-free, or other dietary considerations.

Select Recipes: Choose recipes that pique your interest or suit your dietary preferences. Consider factors such as ingredients availability, cooking time, and complexity. Remember to also select a variety of recipes to ensure a balanced and diverse diet.

Meal Planning: Once you've selected your recipes, plan your meals for the week ahead. Use the provided meal planning guides or templates to organize your breakfasts, lunches, dinners, and snacks. Take note of any ingredients you may need to purchase.

Cook and Enjoy: Follow the step-by-step instructions provided for each recipe to prepare your meals. Enjoy the process of cooking wholesome, nourishing dishes that support your thyroid health. Sit down, savor your meals, and appreciate the journey towards improved well-being with each delicious bite.

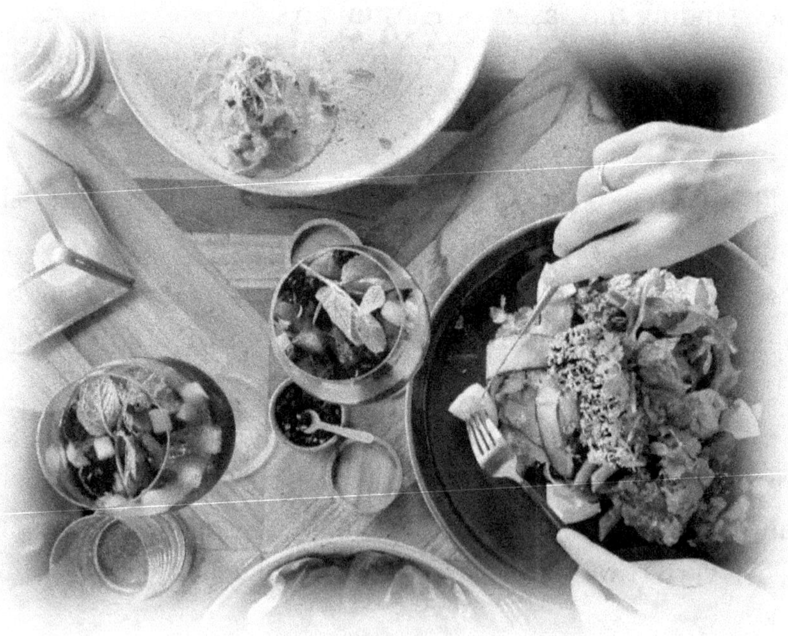

Table of CONTENT

CHAPTER THREE: HEALING RECIPES
LIST OF INGREDIENTS

BREAKFAST RECIPES
Greek Yogurt Parfait with Berries and Almonds
Spinach and Mushroom Omelette
Quinoa Breakfast Bowl with Avocado and Poached Egg
Chia Seed Pudding with Coconut and Mango
Sweet Potato Hash with Turkey Sausage and Eggs
Smoothie Bowl with Spinach, Banana, and Almond Butter
Turmeric Oatmeal with Walnuts and Cinnamon
Salmon and Avocado Toast with Dill Yogurt Sauce
Blueberry Buckwheat Pancakes
Coconut Flour Banana Muffins

SNACKS RECIPES
Greek Yogurt with Berries and Almonds
Avocado and Tomato Rice Cakes
Hummus with Veggie Sticks
Hard-Boiled Eggs with Guacamole
Chia Seed Pudding with Berries
Cottage Cheese and Pineapple Spears
Turkey and Cheese Roll-Ups
Trail Mix with Nuts and Dried Fruit

Apple Slices with Almond Butter
Greek Yogurt Bark with Berries and Almonds

FISH AND SEAFOOD RECIPES

Grilled Salmon with Lemon and Dill
Baked Cod with Tomato and Basil
Shrimp Stir-Fry with Vegetables
Tuna Salad with Avocado and Chickpeas
Salmon and Asparagus Foil Packets
Seared Scallops with Spinach and Garlic Butter
Baked Halibut with Herbed Quinoa
Tuna Lettuce Wraps with Cucumber and Avocado
Shrimp and Vegetable Skewers
Salmon Salad with Lemon Dill Dressing

POULTRY AND MEATS RECIPES

Grilled Chicken with Herbed Quinoa Salad
Turkey Meatballs with Zucchini Noodles
Beef Stir-Fry with Broccoli and Bell Peppers
Baked Chicken Thighs with Sweet Potato Mash
Turkey and Vegetable Skewers with Tzatziki Sauce
Pork Tenderloin with Apple and Sage Sauce
Chicken Curry with Cauliflower Rice
Beef and Vegetable Stir-Fry with Brown Rice
Lemon Herb Roast Chicken with Roasted Vegetables
Spicy Turkey Chili with Beans

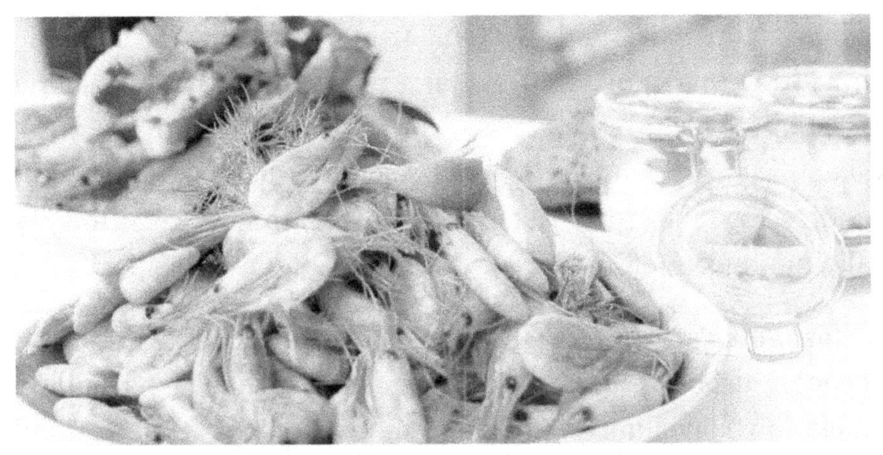

INTRODUCTON

In "Hashimoto's Diet for the Newly Diagnosed," readers embark on a journey of discovery and empowerment through the compelling narrative of a young woman's struggle with Hashimoto's disease. Five years ago, amidst feelings of fatigue and perplexing symptoms, she encountered a pivotal moment when her TPO levels revealed the true identity of her condition — Hashimoto's.

Navigating through the maze of medical consultations, she found solace and guidance from a naturopathic doctor who offered a simple yet profound solution: stay off gluten. This revelation unlocked a path to healing, illuminating the profound connection between autoimmune diseases like Hashimoto's and dietary triggers.

Through the lens of this personal narrative, readers witness the transformative power of dietary interventions in managing Hashimoto's disease. The protagonist's journey from skepticism to conviction underscores the importance of addressing the root cause of illness, rather than merely alleviating symptoms.

"Hashimoto's Diet for the Newly Diagnosed" serves as a beacon of hope and knowledge for individuals embarking on their own healing journeys. With poignant insights and practical advice, this book inspires readers to take control of their health and embrace the transformative potential of a tailored diet.

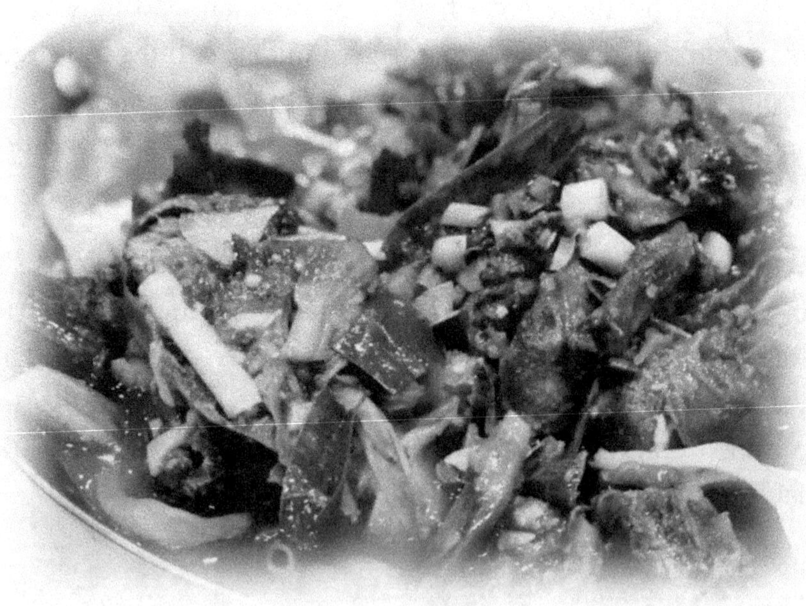

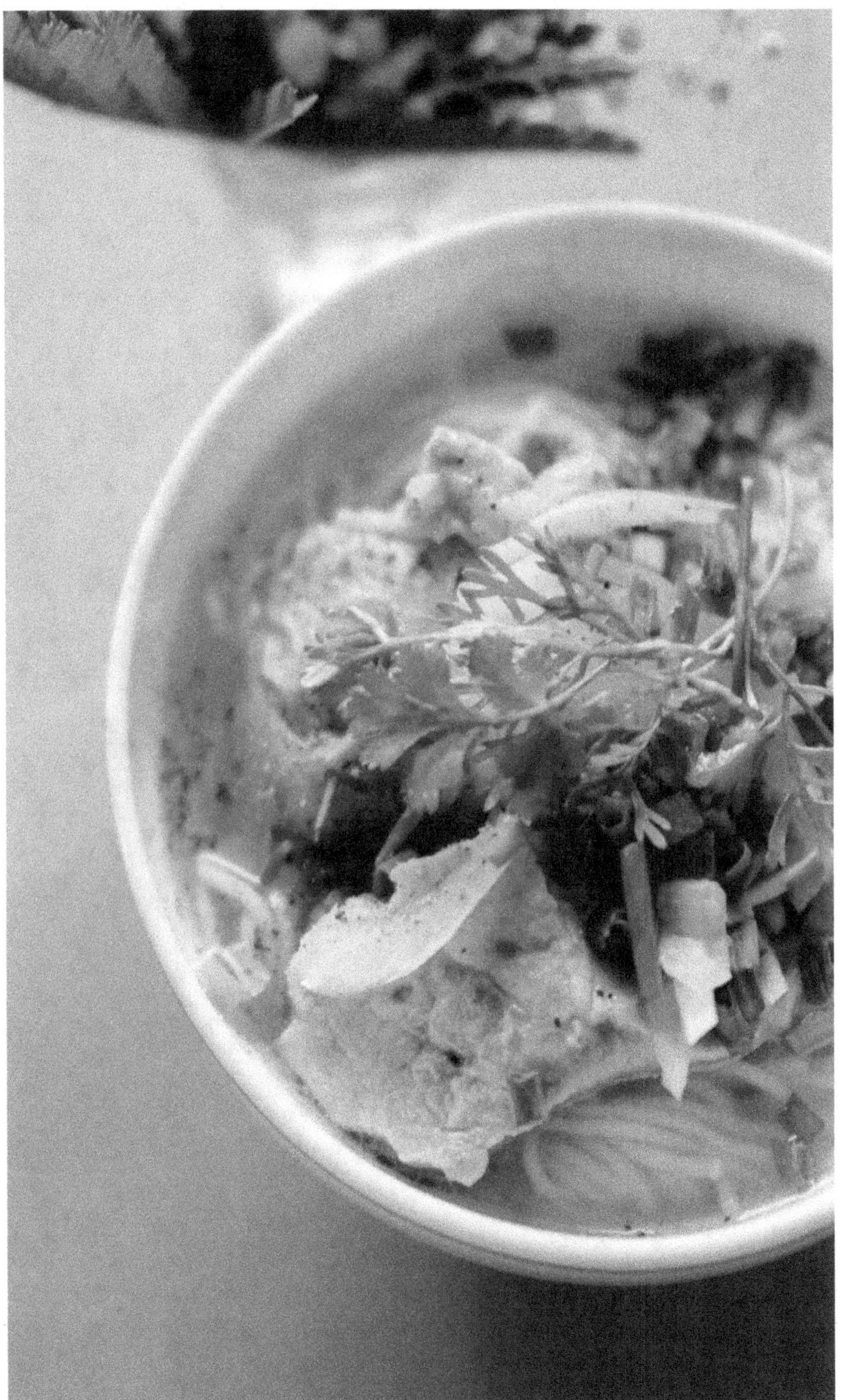

CHAPTER

ONE

OVERVIEW

What is
HASHIMOTO'S

Hashimoto's thyroiditis, also known as chronic lymphocytic thyroiditis, is an autoimmune disorder in which the immune system mistakenly attacks the thyroid gland. This leads to inflammation of the thyroid gland (thyroiditis) and often results in an underactive thyroid (hypothyroidism). It is named after Dr. Hakaru Hashimoto, who first described it in 1912.

Here Are Some Key Points For Someone Newly Diagnosed With Hashimoto's

1. Understanding the Condition: It's important to educate yourself about Hashimoto's thyroiditis. Understanding what it is, how it affects your body, and what to expect can help you better manage the condition.

2. Symptoms: Common symptoms of Hashimoto's include fatigue, weight However, symptoms can vary widely among individuals, and some people may have mild or no symptoms at all.

3. Medical Management: Treatment for Hashimoto's typically involves taking synthetic thyroid hormone medication, such as levothyroxine, to replace

gain, sensitivity to cold, constipation, dry skin, hair loss, and depression.

appropriate dosage based on your symptoms, blood tests, and other factors.

4. Regular Monitoring:
After diagnosis, you'll likely need regular check-ups with your doctor to monitor your thyroid function and adjust medication dosage if necessary. Blood tests to measure thyroid hormone levels (TSH, T3, and T4) are commonly used for monitoring.

5. Lifestyle Factors:
While medication is important, lifestyle factors can also play a role in managing Hashimoto's. Eating a balanced diet, getting regular exercise, managing stress, and getting enough sleep can all help support thyroid health.

the hormones that your thyroid is not producing enough of. Your doctor will determine the

immune system imbalances. This may involve working with a healthcare provider to identify and address potential triggers such as food sensitivities, gut health issues, or environmental toxins.

7. Support: Connecting
with others who have Hashimoto's can provide valuable support and insights. There are many online communities, support groups, and forums where you can connect with others who understand what you're going through.

8. Long-Term Outlook:
With proper management, most people with Hashimoto's can lead normal, healthy lives. However, it's important to stay vigilant about

6. Autoimmune Management: Since Hashimoto's is an autoimmune disorder, some people find relief from symptoms by addressing underlying monitoring your thyroid function and addressing any changes in symptoms with your healthcare provider.

DIAGNOSIS OF HASHIMOTO'S THYROIDITIS

Upon receiving a diagnosis of Hashimoto's thyroiditis, understanding the relationship between diet and managing symptoms becomes crucial. A Hashimoto's diet aims to support thyroid function, reduce inflammation, and alleviate symptoms associated with the condition. For individuals newly diagnosed with Hashimoto's, adopting a diet tailored to their needs can significantly improve their quality of life. This dietary approach often draws from the principles outlined in Hashimoto's diet cookbooks, which provide guidance on selecting foods that promote thyroid health and minimizing those that may exacerbate symptoms.

Hashimoto's diet cookbooks typically emphasize whole, nutrient-dense foods while avoiding or limiting potential triggers for inflammation and immune system dysfunction. *Here's a breakdown of key dietary recommendations commonly found in these cookbooks:*

1. Gluten-Free: Many individuals with Hashimoto's find relief from symptoms by eliminating gluten from their diet. Gluten, a protein found in wheat, barley, and rye, can trigger inflammation and exacerbate autoimmune responses in some people. Hashimoto's diet cookbooks often feature gluten-free recipes using alternative grains like rice, quinoa, and gluten-free oats.

2. Low Inflammatory Foods: Foods with anti-inflammatory properties are often prioritized in Hashimoto's diets. This includes fresh fruits and vegetables, fatty fish rich in omega-3 fatty acids (such as salmon and mackerel), nuts, seeds, and healthy fats like olive oil and avocado. These foods can help reduce inflammation and support immune system balance.

3. Balanced Macronutrients: A well-rounded diet that includes adequate protein, healthy fats, and complex carbohydrates is essential for supporting thyroid function and overall health. Hashimoto's diet cookbooks provide recipes that incorporate a balance of macronutrients, ensuring individuals receive the nutrients needed for optimal thyroid function and energy levels.

4. Limiting Goitrogens: Some foods contain compounds known as goitrogens, which can interfere with thyroid function when consumed in large amounts. These include cruciferous vegetables like broccoli, cauliflower, and cabbage, as well as soy-based products. While small amounts of goitrogenic foods are generally safe for most people, Hashimoto's diet cookbooks often suggest consuming them in moderation or cooking them to reduce their goitrogenic properties.

5. Individualized Approach: It's important to recognize that there is no one-size-fits-all approach to diet for Hashimoto's. Each person may have unique dietary triggers and sensitivities. Hashimoto's diet cookbooks encourage experimentation and self-awareness, empowering individuals to identify which foods support their health and which may exacerbate symptoms.

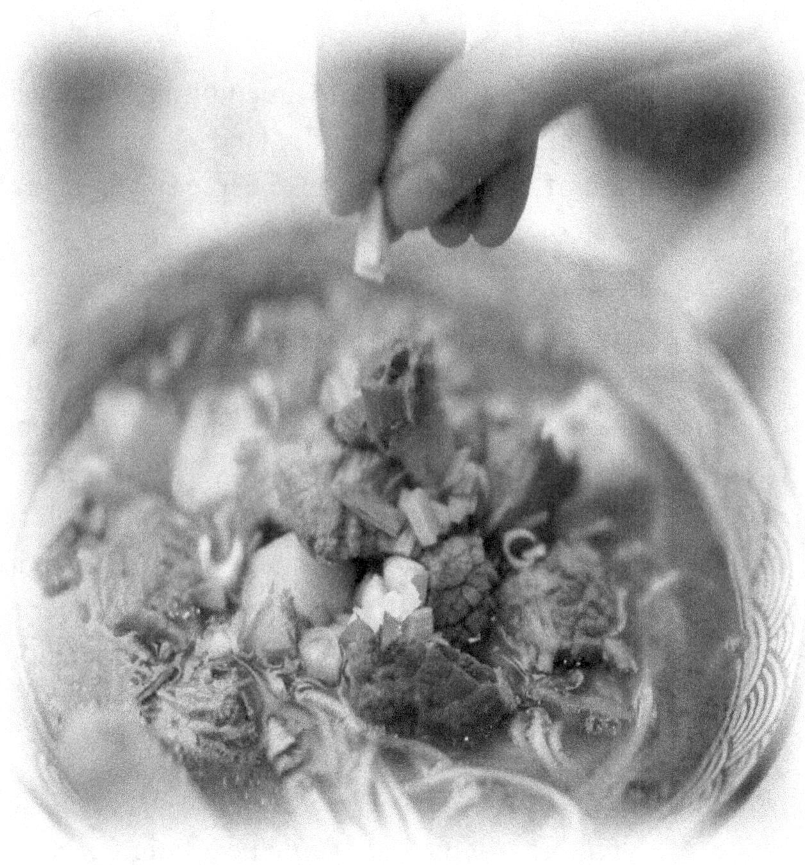

OVERVIEW Of HASHIMOTO'S THYROIDITIS

- **Type:** Hashimoto's thyroiditis is an autoimmune disease that primarily affects the thyroid gland. It is the most common cause of hypothyroidism (underactive thyroid) in the United States.

- **Causes:** The exact cause of Hashimoto's thyroiditis is not fully understood, but it is believed to result from a combination of genetic predisposition and environmental triggers. In Hashimoto's, the immune system mistakenly attacks the thyroid gland, leading to inflammation and damage to thyroid tissue. Factors such as genetics, hormonal imbalances, excessive iodine intake, and certain viral infections may contribute to the development of Hashimoto's.

- **Symptoms:** Hashimoto's thyroiditis can cause a wide range of symptoms, which may include fatigue, weight gain, constipation, dry skin, hair loss, sensitivity to cold, muscle weakness, joint pain, depression, and menstrual irregularities. However, some individuals with Hashimoto's may experience few or no symptoms, especially in the early stages of the disease.

- **Preventive Measures:** While there is no known way to prevent Hashimoto's thyroiditis, certain lifestyle factors may help reduce the risk of developing complications or worsening symptoms. These include maintaining a healthy diet, managing stress levels, getting regular exercise, avoiding smoking, and minimizing exposure to environmental toxins.

- **Treatment:** Treatment for Hashimoto's thyroiditis typically involves medication to replace the hormones that the thyroid gland is no longer producing enough of. The most common medication prescribed is synthetic thyroid hormone (such as levothyroxine), which helps restore normal thyroid function and alleviate symptoms of hypothyroidism. The dosage of thyroid hormone medication is adjusted based on regular blood tests to monitor thyroid hormone levels.

In addition to medication, other treatment options for Hashimoto's may include:

Monitoring: Regular monitoring of thyroid function through blood tests is essential to ensure that hormone levels are within the target range and adjust medication dosage as needed.

Dietary Changes: Some individuals may benefit from dietary modifications, such as avoiding gluten and reducing consumption of goitrogenic foods (e.g., cruciferous vegetables) that may interfere with thyroid function.

Supplements: Certain supplements, such as selenium and vitamin D, may help support thyroid health and reduce inflammation in individuals with Hashimoto's. However, it's essential to consult with a healthcare provider before starting any new supplements.

Managing Stress: Stress management techniques, such as meditation, yoga, and deep breathing exercises, may help reduce inflammation and improve overall well-being in individuals with Hashimoto's.

Supportive Therapies: In some cases, complementary and alternative therapies, such as acupuncture, may provide symptom relief and support immune system function.

Overall, treatment for Hashimoto's thyroiditis aims to alleviate symptoms, restore thyroid function, and improve quality of life for affected individuals. It is essential for individuals with Hashimoto's to work closely with their healthcare providers to develop a personalized treatment plan tailored to their specific needs and symptoms.

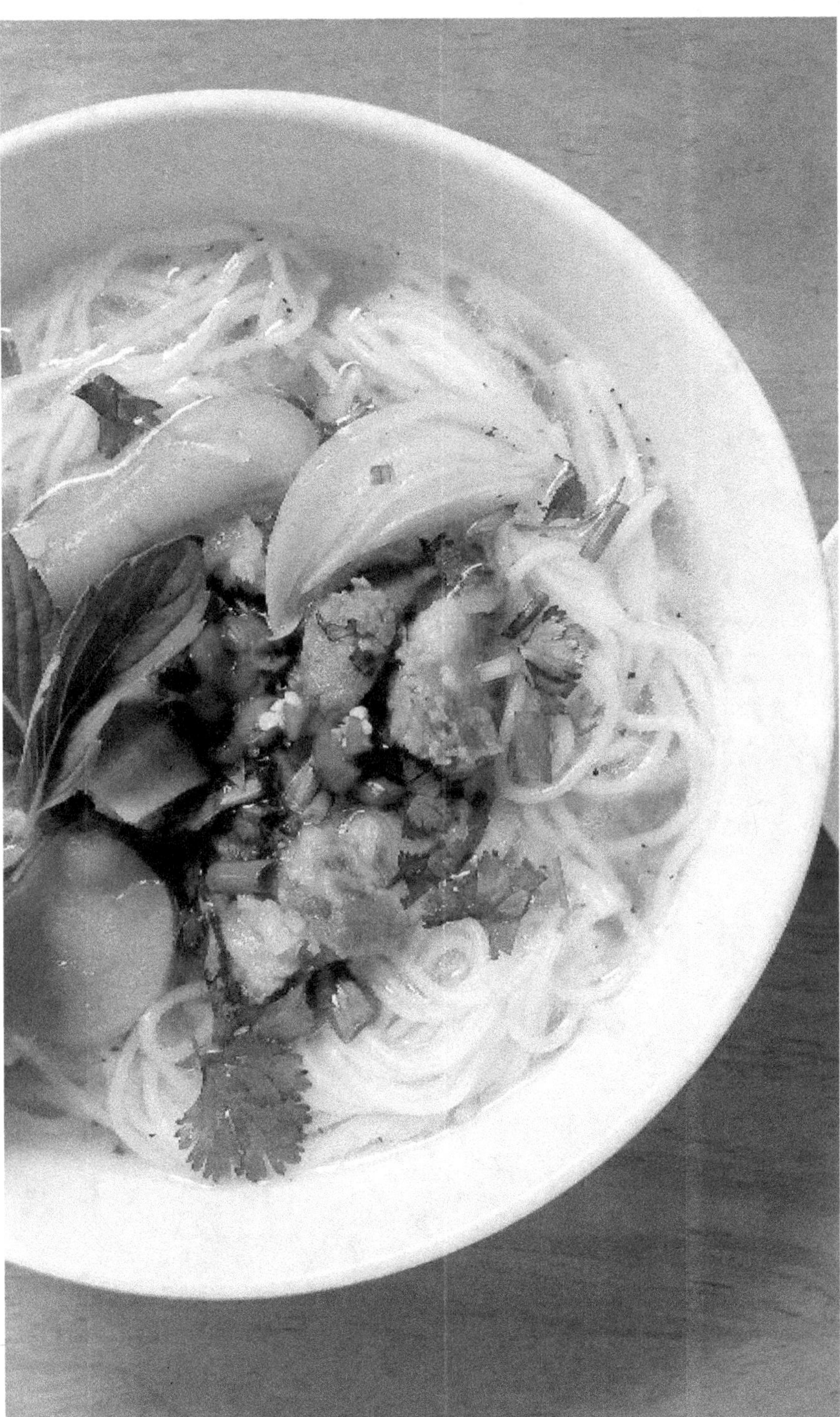

CHAPTER

TWO

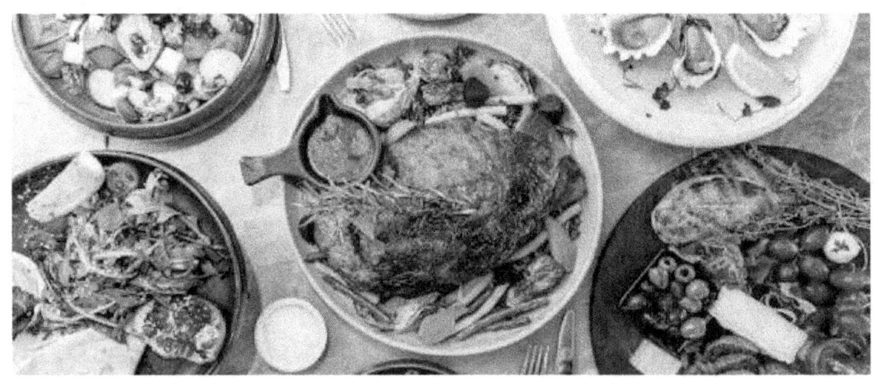

IMPACT OF HASHIMOTO'S ON THE THYROID

Hashimoto's thyroiditis has a significant impact on the thyroid gland, leading to various changes and disruptions in its structure and function. Here are some of the key effects of Hashimoto's on the thyroid:

1. **Thyroid Inflammation:** Hashimoto's thyroiditis is characterized by chronic inflammation of the thyroid gland. This inflammation can lead to swelling and enlargement of the thyroid, a condition known as goiter. Over time, the ongoing inflammation can damage thyroid tissue and impair its ability to produce hormones.

2. **Hypothyroidism:** The primary consequence of Hashimoto's thyroiditis is hypothyroidism, or an underactive thyroid. As the autoimmune attack on the thyroid gland progresses, it gradually impairs the gland's ability to produce thyroid hormones—triiodothyronine (T3) and thyroxine (T4).

This deficiency in thyroid hormone production leads to a slowdown in metabolic processes throughout the body, resulting in symptoms such as fatigue, weight gain, cold intolerance, and constipation.

3. Thyroid Dysfunction: Hashimoto's thyroiditis can cause fluctuations in thyroid hormone levels, leading to periods of hyperthyroidism (an overactive thyroid) followed by hypothyroidism. This pattern, known as Hashitoxicosis, occurs as a result of thyroid cell destruction releasing stored thyroid hormones into the bloodstream.

4. Autoimmune Attack: Hashimoto's thyroiditis is an autoimmune disease, meaning the body's immune system mistakenly attacks its tissues. In the case of Hashimoto's, the immune system targets the thyroid gland, causing damage and dysfunction. This autoimmune attack can result in the formation of thyroid antibodies, such as thyroid peroxidase antibodies (TPOAb) and thyroglobulin antibodies (TgAb), which are often detected in blood tests for Hashimoto's.

5. Thyroid Nodules: In some cases, Hashimoto's thyroiditis may be associated with the development of thyroid nodules—abnormal growths or lumps within the thyroid gland. While most thyroid nodules are benign, some may be cancerous. Regular monitoring and evaluation by a healthcare provider are essential to assess the risk of thyroid nodules and determine appropriate management.

BENEFITS OF HASHIMOTO'S DIET

Adopting a diet tailored to Hashimoto's thyroiditis can offer several potential benefits for individuals with the condition. While dietary changes may not cure Hashimoto's or eliminate the need for medication, they can help manage symptoms, support thyroid health, and improve overall well-being. Here are some potential benefits of a Hashimoto's diet:

1. **Reduced Inflammation**: Many Hashimoto's diets focus on reducing inflammation, which is a key factor in autoimmune diseases like Hashimoto's thyroiditis. By avoiding inflammatory foods and emphasizing anti-inflammatory foods such as fruits, vegetables, fatty fish, and healthy fats, individuals may experience

2. **Support for Thyroid Function:** Certain nutrients are essential for thyroid health, including iodine, selenium, zinc, and vitamin D. A Hashimoto's diet often includes foods rich in these nutrients to support thyroid function and hormone production. For example, seafood, Brazil nuts, dairy products, and fortified foods are excellent sources of iodine and selenium, while fatty fish, nuts, seeds, and eggs provide omega-3 fatty acids, zinc, and vitamin D.

3. **Stabilized Blood Sugar Levels:** Blood sugar fluctuations can impact energy levels and mood, which are common concerns for individuals with Hashimoto's. A diet

a decrease in overall inflammation levels.

fruits, vegetables, whole grains, lean proteins, and healthy fats—can help stabilize blood sugar levels and provide sustained energy throughout the day.

4. Improved Gut Health: There is growing evidence to suggest that gut health plays a role in autoimmune conditions like Hashimoto's thyroiditis. Certain dietary factors, such as gluten, dairy, and processed foods, may contribute to gut inflammation and dysbiosis (imbalance of gut bacteria). By eliminating potential trigger foods and incorporating gut-supportive foods like probiotics, prebiotics, and fermented foods, individuals may experience improvements in digestive health and immune function.

rich in whole, nutrient-dense foods—such as Hashimoto's thyroiditis. A Hashimoto's diet that emphasizes whole, nutrient-dense foods and balances macronutrients can support healthy weight management by promoting satiety, reducing cravings, and stabilizing metabolism.

6. Reduced Symptom Severity: While dietary changes may not eliminate symptoms entirely, many individuals with Hashimoto's report improvements in symptoms such as fatigue, brain fog, joint pain, and mood disturbances after adopting a Hashimoto's diet. Identifying and avoiding trigger foods, managing nutrient deficiencies, and supporting overall health can contribute to symptom

5. Weight Management: Weight gain and difficulty losing weight are common symptoms of hypothyroidism, which often accompanies

HOW DIET AFFECT HASHIMOTO'S DISEASE

1. Inflammation: Certain foods can contribute to inflammation in the body, which may exacerbate autoimmune responses in individuals with Hashimoto's. Chronic inflammation can worsen thyroid gland damage and impair thyroid function. Processed foods, refined sugars, trans fats, and excess omega-6 fatty acids found in vegetable oils are examples of dietary factors that can promote

relief and improved quality of life.

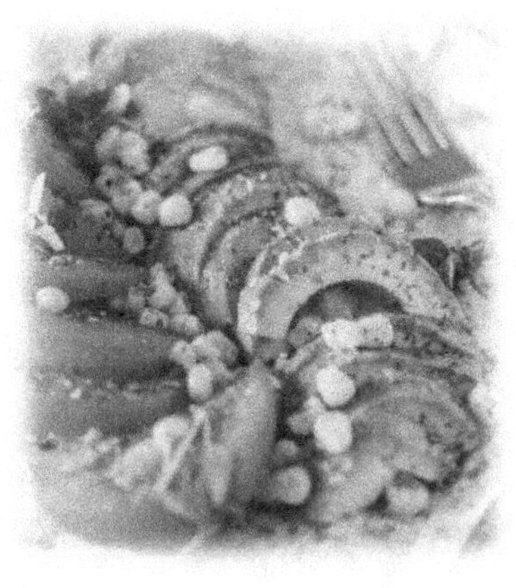

inflammation and alleviate symptoms.

2. Gut Health: Emerging research suggests a link between gut health and autoimmune diseases like Hashimoto's thyroiditis. The gut microbiota play a crucial role in regulating immune function, and imbalances in gut bacteria (dysbiosis) may contribute to autoimmune dysfunction. Certain dietary factors, such as

inflammation. Conversely, a diet rich in anti-inflammatory foods such as fruits, vegetables, fatty fish, nuts, seeds, and olive oil may help reduce responses. Eliminating or reducing these trigger foods and incorporating gut-supportive foods like probiotics, prebiotics, and fermented foods may help promote a healthy gut microbiome and reduce autoimmune activity.

3. Nutrient Deficiencies: Nutrient deficiencies can impact thyroid function and exacerbate symptoms of Hashimoto's thyroiditis. Key nutrients for thyroid health include iodine, selenium, zinc, iron, vitamin D, and B vitamins. A diet lacking in these nutrients may impair thyroid hormone

gluten and dairy, have been implicated in gut inflammation and permeability (leaky gut), potentially triggering or exacerbating autoimmune seafood, dairy products, and iodized salt are essential for thyroid hormone synthesis, while selenium-rich foods like Brazil nuts, seafood, and organ meats help regulate thyroid function and reduce inflammation.

4. Gluten Sensitivity: Some individuals with Hashimoto's thyroiditis may have gluten sensitivity or celiac disease, which can exacerbate autoimmune responses and thyroid inflammation. Gluten, a protein found in wheat, barley, and rye, has been implicated in triggering autoimmune diseases and may contribute to gut

production and contribute to hypothyroidism. Conversely, consuming a balanced diet rich in nutrient-dense foods can help support thyroid function and alleviate symptoms. For example, iodine-rich foods like symptoms, and improve overall well-being.

5. Blood Sugar Regulation: Imbalances in blood sugar levels can affect energy levels, mood, and hormone regulation, all of which are concerns for individuals with Hashimoto's thyroiditis. Consuming refined carbohydrates, sugary foods, and processed snacks can lead to rapid spikes and crashes in blood sugar levels, exacerbating fatigue and mood swings. A diet rich in complex carbohydrates, fiber,

protein, and healthy fats helps stabilize blood sugar levels, providing sustained energy and mood stability.

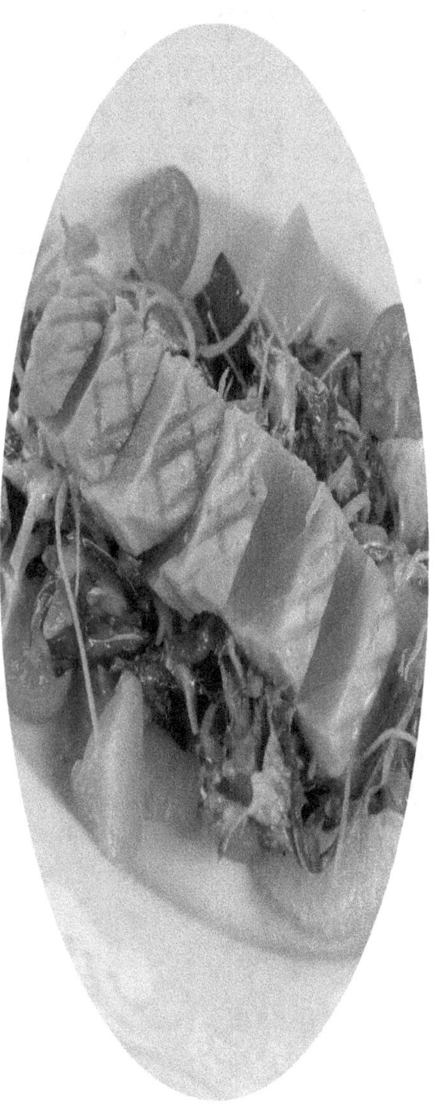

TIPS TO ACHIEVE OPTIMAL HEALTH WITH HASHIMOTO'S DIET

When it comes to managing Hashimoto's thyroiditis through diet, understanding which foods to include and which to avoid is crucial for achieving optimum health. A Hashimoto's diet cookbook tailored for newly diagnosed individuals can provide valuable guidance on selecting foods that support thyroid function, reduce inflammation, and alleviate symptoms.

Here's a comprehensive overview of foods to eat and avoid on a Hashimoto's diet:

FOODS TO EAT

1. Whole, Nutrient-Dense Foods: Emphasize whole, unprocessed foods rich in nutrients essential for thyroid health, such as iodine, selenium, zinc, and vitamin D. Include plenty of fruits, vegetables, lean proteins, whole grains, nuts, seeds, and healthy fats in your diet.

Incorporate iodine-rich foods such as seafood (e.g., fish, shellfish), seaweed, dairy products, and iodized salt into your meals to support thyroid function.

3. Selenium-Rich Foods: Selenium helps regulate thyroid hormone metabolism and reduce inflammation. Include

2. Iodine-Rich Foods:
Iodine is a crucial nutrient for thyroid hormone synthesis.
tuna, shrimp), organ meats (e.g., liver), eggs, and whole grains in your diet to support thyroid health.

4. Omega-3 Fatty Acids:
Omega-3 fatty acids have anti-inflammatory properties and may help reduce autoimmune activity in Hashimoto's thyroiditis. Consume fatty fish (e.g., salmon, mackerel, sardines), flaxseeds, chia seeds, walnuts, and algae oil to incorporate omega-3s into your diet.

5.Antioxidant-Rich Foods: Antioxidants help protect thyroid tissue from damage caused by oxidative stress and inflammation. Include a variety of antioxidant-rich foods such as berries, citrus fruits, leafy greens, carrots, sweet potatoes, tomatoes, and nuts to support thyroid health.

selenium-rich foods like Brazil nuts, seafood (e.g.,

6. Probiotic Foods:
Probiotics help maintain a healthy gut microbiome and support immune function, which is important for individuals with autoimmune conditions like Hashimoto's. Incorporate probiotic-rich foods such as yogurt, kefir, sauerkraut, kimchi, and kombucha into your diet to promote gut health.

7. Gluten-Free Grains:
Some individuals with Hashimoto's thyroiditis may benefit from avoiding gluten-containing grains like wheat, barley, and rye, as gluten sensitivity can exacerbate autoimmune responses and thyroid inflammation. Opt for gluten-free grains such as rice, quinoa, millet, buckwheat, and gluten-free oats instead.

FOODS TO AVOID

1. Gluten: Gluten, a protein found in wheat, barley, and rye, has been implicated in triggering autoimmune reactions and exacerbating thyroid inflammation in some individuals with Hashimoto's. Avoid gluten-containing foods such as bread, pasta, cereals, baked goods, and processed snacks.

2. Processed and Refined Foods: Processed foods high in refined sugars, unhealthy fats, additives, and preservatives can promote inflammation and disrupt gut health. Limit or avoid processed snacks, sugary beverages, fast food, fried foods, and packaged convenience foods.

3. Goitrogenic Foods: Goitrogens are compounds found in certain foods that individuals with Hashimoto's may benefit from cooking or steaming goitrogenic foods to reduce their goitrogenic properties. Examples of goitrogenic foods include cruciferous vegetables (e.g., broccoli, cauliflower, cabbage, kale), soy-based products, peanuts, and millet.

4. Excessive Iodine: While iodine is essential for thyroid health, excessive iodine intake can exacerbate thyroid inflammation and worsen symptoms in individuals with Hashimoto's. Avoid excessive iodine supplementation and limit intake of iodine-rich foods if recommended by a healthcare provider.

5. Alcohol and Caffeine: Alcohol and caffeine consumption can disrupt

can interfere with thyroid function by inhibiting iodine uptake or thyroid hormone synthesis. While goitrogens are generally safe when consumed in moderation, consumption from sources like coffee, tea, and energy drinks.

6. Artificial Sweeteners and Additives:

Artificial sweeteners, flavorings, colorings, and preservatives found in processed foods and beverages can trigger hormone balance, interfere with sleep quality, and exacerbate symptoms of Hashimoto's thyroiditis. Limit alcohol intake and moderate caffeine inflammatory responses and exacerbate symptoms in some individuals with Hashimoto's. Opt for whole, minimally processed foods and natural sweeteners like honey, maple syrup, or stevia instead.

THREE

HEALING RECIPES

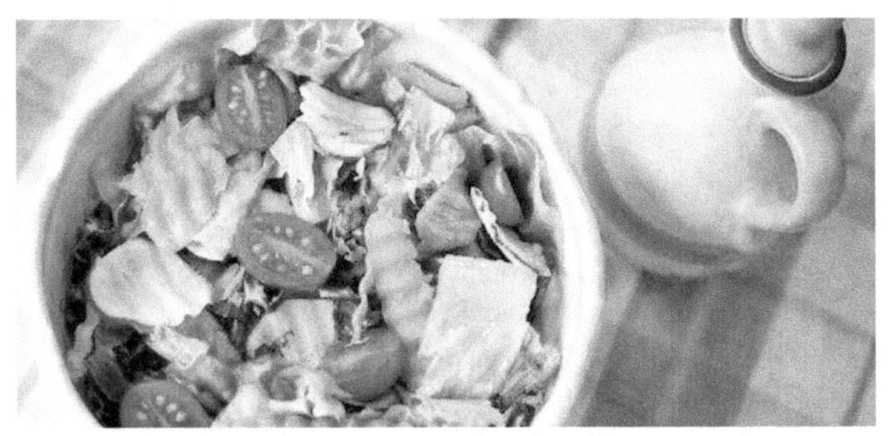

SHOPPING LIST

Whole Grains and Lean Proteins

Gluten-Free Options

Quinoa: A complete protein and gluten-free grain.

Brown rice: Rich in fiber and nutrients, suitable for a gluten-free diet.

Gluten-free pasta: Made from alternative flours such as rice or chickpea flour.

Oats (certified gluten-free): Provide fiber and may help regulate blood sugar levels.

Poultry (chicken, turkey): Choose organic, free-range options when possible.

Fish (salmon, mackerel, sardines): Rich in omega-3 fatty acids, which may help reduce inflammation.

Lean cuts of beef or pork: Opt for grass-fed or pasture-raised options.

Legumes (lentils, black beans, chickpeas): Good plant-based protein sources.

Leafy greens (spinach, kale, Swiss chard): Rich in vitamins, minerals, and antioxidants.

Cruciferous vegetables (broccoli, cauliflower, **Brussels sprouts):** Contains compounds that may support thyroid function when cooked.

Colorful vegetables (bell peppers, carrots, tomatoes): Provide a variety of nutrients and antioxidants.

Avocado: A source of healthy fats and potassium.

Berries (blueberries, strawberries, raspberries): Rich in antioxidants and fiber.

Citrus fruits (lemons, oranges): High in vitamin C and add flavor to dishes.

Garlic and onions: Offer flavor and potential health benefits.

Dairy Alternatives

Unsweetened almond milk, coconut milk, or oat milk: Suitable alternatives to cow's milk.

Dairy-free yogurt or cheese: Made from plant-based sources such as coconut or almond milk.

Healthy Fats

Olive oil: A source of monounsaturated fats and antioxidants.

Coconut oil: Contains medium-chain triglycerides (MCTs) which may support thyroid health.

Avocado oil: High in monounsaturated fats and suitable for high-heat cooking.

Nuts and seeds (almonds, walnuts, chia seeds, flaxseeds): Provide healthy fats, protein, and fiber.

Herbs and Spices

Turmeric: Contains curcumin, which may have anti-inflammatory properties.
Ginger: Supports digestion and may reduce inflammation.
Cinnamon: Helps stabilize blood sugar levels.
Fresh herbs (parsley, **cilantro, basil):** Add flavor and provide antioxidants.

Miscellaneous

Apple cider vinegar: May support digestion and blood sugar regulation.
Sea salt or Himalayan pink salt: Provides minerals and enhances flavor.
Herbal teas: Choose caffeine-free options such as peppermint or chamomile.

Breakfast

recipes

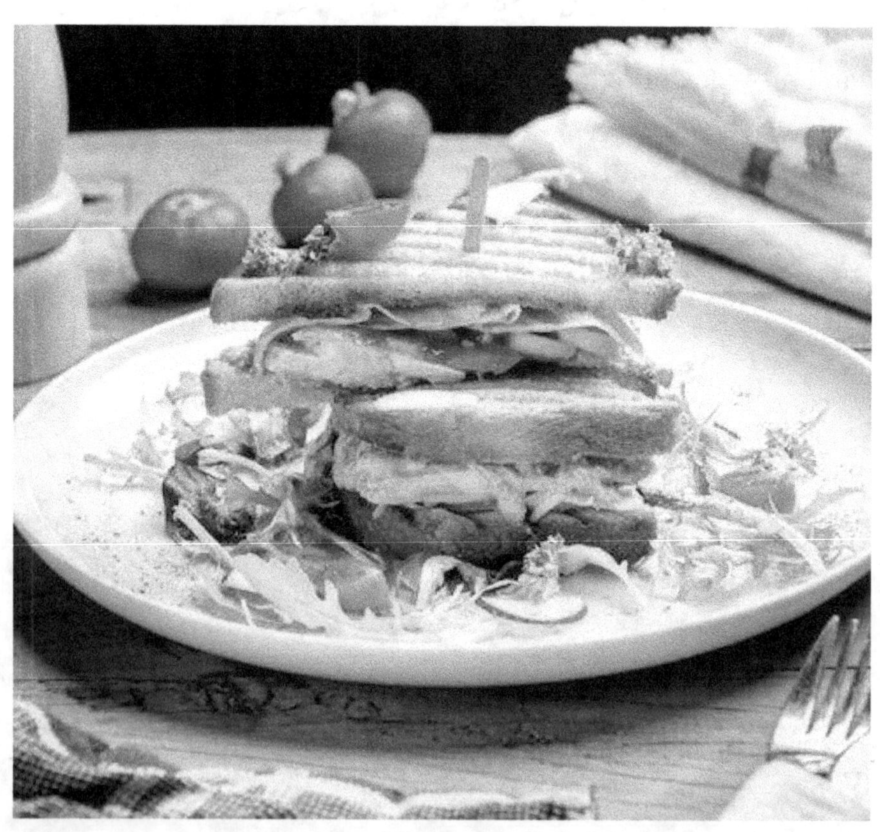

GREEK YOGURT PARFAIT WITH BERRIES AND ALMONDS

INGREDIENTS

- ❖ Greek yogurt (1 cup)
- ❖ Mixed berries (1/2 cup)
- ❖ Almonds (1/4 cup, chopped)
- ❖ Honey or maple syrup (optional, for sweetness)

INSTUCTIONS

1. In a serving bowl or glass, layer Greek yogurt, mixed berries, and chopped almonds.
2. Drizzle with honey or maple syrup if desired.
3. Serve immediately and enjoy this protein-rich breakfast.

SPINACH AND MUSHROOM OMELETTE

INGREDIENTS

- ❖ Spinach (1 cup, chopped)
- ❖ Mushrooms (1/2 cup, sliced)
- ❖ Onion (1/4 cup, diced)
- ❖ Olive oil (1 tbsp)
- ❖ Salt and pepper to taste

INSTUCTIONS

1. In a skillet, heat olive oil over medium heat.
2. Add diced onion and sliced mushrooms, and cook until softened.
3. Add chopped spinach to the skillet and cook until wilted.
4. In a bowl, beat eggs and season with salt and pepper.
5. Pour the beaten eggs over the vegetables in the skillet and cook until set.
6. Fold the omelette in half and transfer to a plate.
7. Serve hot and enjoy this nutritious breakfast.

QUINOA BREAKFAST BOWL WITH AVOCADO AND POACHED

INGREDIENTS

- ❖ Quinoa (1/2 cup, cooked)
- ❖ Avocado (1/2, sliced)
- ❖ Poached egg (1)
- ❖ Cherry tomatoes (1/4 cup, halved)
- ❖ Fresh cilantro or parsley (1 tbsp, chopped)
- ❖ Olive oil (1 tbsp)
- ❖ Lemon juice (1 tbsp)
- ❖ Salt and pepper to taste

INSTUCTIONS

1. In a bowl, layer cooked quinoa, sliced avocado, halved cherry tomatoes, and poached egg.
2. Drizzle with olive oil and lemon juice.
3. Season with salt, pepper, and chopped cilantro or parsley.
4. Serve immediately and enjoy this protein-packed breakfast.

CHIA SEED PUDDING WITH COCONUT AND MANGO

INGREDIENTS

- ❖ Chia seeds (3 tbsp)
- ❖ Coconut milk (1 cup)
- ❖ Mango (1/2, diced)
- ❖ Shredded coconut (2 tbsp)
- ❖ Honey or maple syrup (optional, for sweetness)

INSTUCTIONS

1. In a bowl, mix chia seeds and coconut milk.
2. Let the mixture sit for 1015 minutes until thickened.
3. Stir in diced mango and shredded coconut.
4. Sweeten with honey or maple syrup if desired.
5. Divide the chia seed pudding into serving cups and refrigerate for at least 1 hour.
6. Serve chilled and enjoy this refreshing breakfast.

SWEET POTATO HASH WITH TURKEY SAUSAGE AND EGGS

INGREDIENTS

- Sweet potato (1, diced)
- Turkey sausage (2 links, sliced)
- Bell pepper (1/2, diced)
- Onion (1/4, diced)
- Garlic (1 clove, minced)
- Olive oil (1 tbsp)
- Eggs (2)
- Salt and pepper to taste

INSTUCTIONS

1. In a skillet, heat olive oil over medium heat.
2. Add diced sweet potato to the skillet and cook until softened and lightly browned.
3. Add sliced turkey sausage, diced bell pepper, diced onion, and minced garlic to the skillet. Cook until vegetables are tender and sausage is cooked through.
4. Season with salt and pepper to taste.
5. In a separate skillet, fry eggs to desired doneness.
6. Serve sweet potato hash topped with fried eggs.
7. Enjoy this hearty and satisfying breakfast.

SMOOTHIE BOWL WITH SPINACH, BANANA, AND

INGREDIENTS

- ❖ Spinach (1 cup)
- ❖ Banana (1, frozen)
- ❖ Almond butter (2 tbsp)
- ❖ Almond milk (1/2 cup)
- ❖ Chia seeds (1 tbsp)
- ❖ Fresh berries (for topping)
- ❖ Granola (for topping)

INSTUCTIONS

1. In a blender, combine spinach, frozen banana, almond butter, almond milk, and chia seeds.
2. Blend until smooth and creamy.
3. Pour the smoothie into a bowl.
4. Top with fresh berries and granola.
5. Serve immediately and enjoy this nutrient-packed breakfast.

TURMERIC OATMEAL WITH WALNUTS AND CINNAMON

INGREDIENTS

- ❖ Rolled oats (1/2 cup)
- ❖ Turmeric powder (1/2 tsp)
- ❖ Cinnamon (1/2 tsp)
- ❖ Walnuts (2 tbsp, chopped)
- ❖ Maple syrup or honey (1 tbsp, optional, for sweetness)
- ❖ Almond milk (1 cup)

INSTUCTIONS

1. In a saucepan, combine rolled oats, turmeric powder, cinnamon, chopped walnuts, and almond milk.
2. Cook over medium heat, stirring occasionally, until oats are cooked and the mixture thickens.
3. Sweeten with maple syrup or honey if desired.
4. Serve hot and enjoy this warm and comforting breakfast.

SALMON AND AVOCADO TOAST WITH DILL YOGURT SAUCE

INGREDIENTS

- ❖ Whole grain bread (2 slices, toasted)
- ❖ Smoked salmon (2 oz)
- ❖ Avocado (1/2, sliced)
- ❖ Greek yogurt (2 tbsp)
- ❖ Fresh dill (1 tbsp, chopped)
- ❖ Lemon juice (1 tsp)
- ❖ Salt and pepper to taste

INSTUCTIONS

1. In a small bowl, mix Greek yogurt, chopped dill, lemon juice, salt, and pepper to make the dill yogurt sauce.
2. Spread the dill yogurt sauce on toasted whole grain bread slices.
3. Top with sliced avocado and smoked salmon.
4. Serve immediately and enjoy this protein-rich breakfast.

BLUEBERRY BUCKWHEAT PANCAKES

INGREDIENTS

- ❖ Buckwheat flour (1 cup)
- ❖ Baking powder (1 tsp)
- ❖ Almond milk (1 cup)
- ❖ Egg (1)
- ❖ Blueberries (1/2 cup)
- ❖ Maple syrup (for serving)

INSTUCTIONS

1. In a bowl, whisk together buckwheat flour and baking powder.
2. Add almond milk and egg to the flour mixture and whisk until smooth.
3. Gently fold in blueberries.
4. Heat a skillet or griddle over medium heat and lightly grease with oil.
5. Pour pancake batter onto the skillet to form pancakes.
6. Cook until bubbles form on the surface, then flip and cook until golden brown on the other side.
7. Serve warm with maple syrup and enjoy these hearty and nutritious pancakes.

COCONUT FLOUR BANANA MUFFINS

INGREDIENTS

- ❖ Coconut flour (1/2 cup)
- ❖ Ripe bananas (2, mashed)
- ❖ Eggs (2)
- ❖ Coconut oil (2 tbsp, melted)
- ❖ Maple syrup (2 tbsp, optional, for sweetness)
- ❖ Baking powder (1/2 tsp)
- ❖ Vanilla extract (1/2 tsp)
- ❖ Cinnamon (1/2 tsp)

INSTUCTIONS

1. Preheat the oven to 350°F (175°C) and line a muffin tin with paper liners.
2. In a bowl, combine mashed bananas, eggs, melted coconut oil, maple syrup (if using), vanilla extract, and cinnamon. Mix until well combined.
3. Add coconut flour and baking powder to the wet ingredients and stir until smooth.
4. Divide the batter evenly among the muffin cups.
5. Bake for 2025 minutes or until a toothpick inserted into the center comes out clean.
6. Allow the muffins to cool slightly before serving.

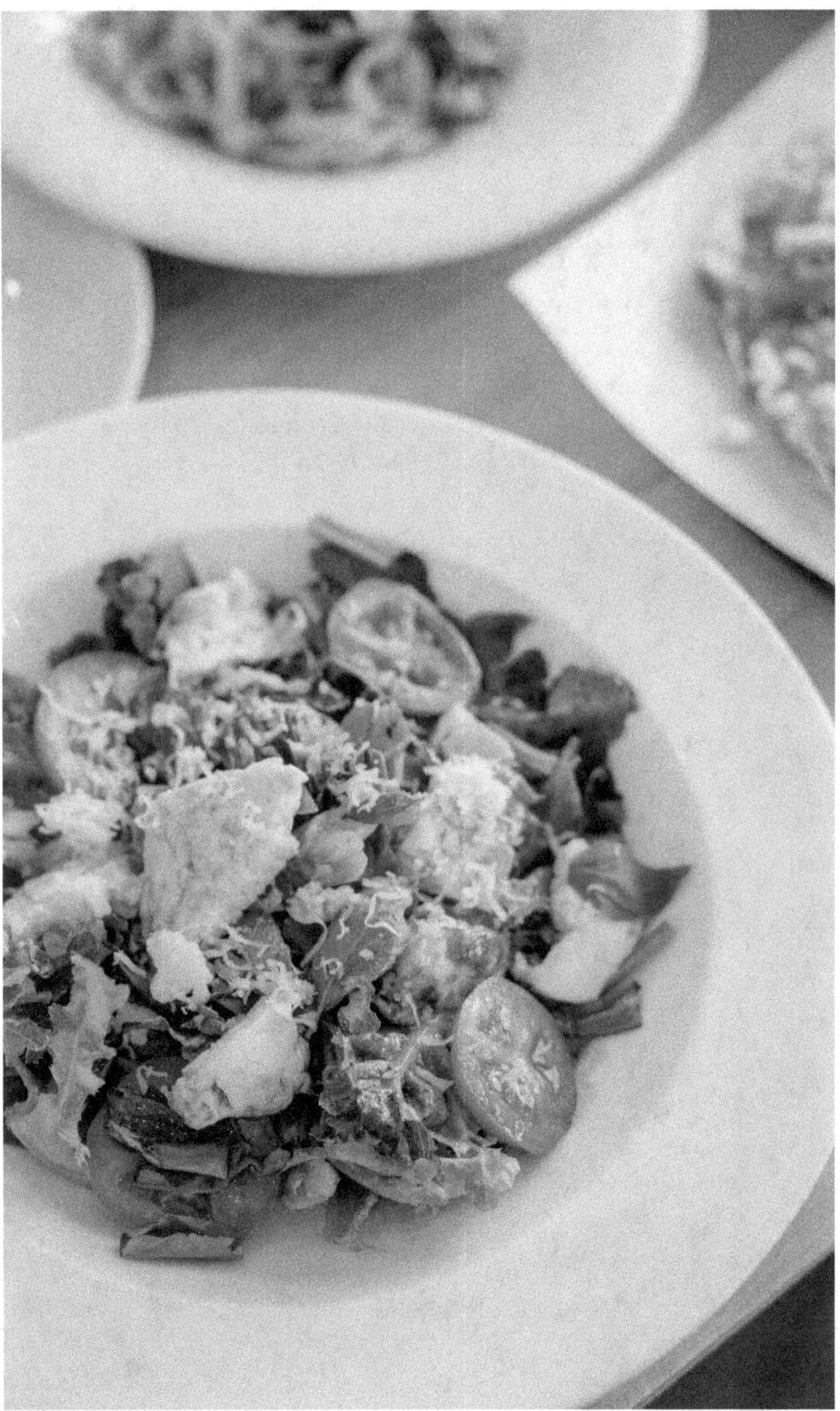

Snacks

recipes

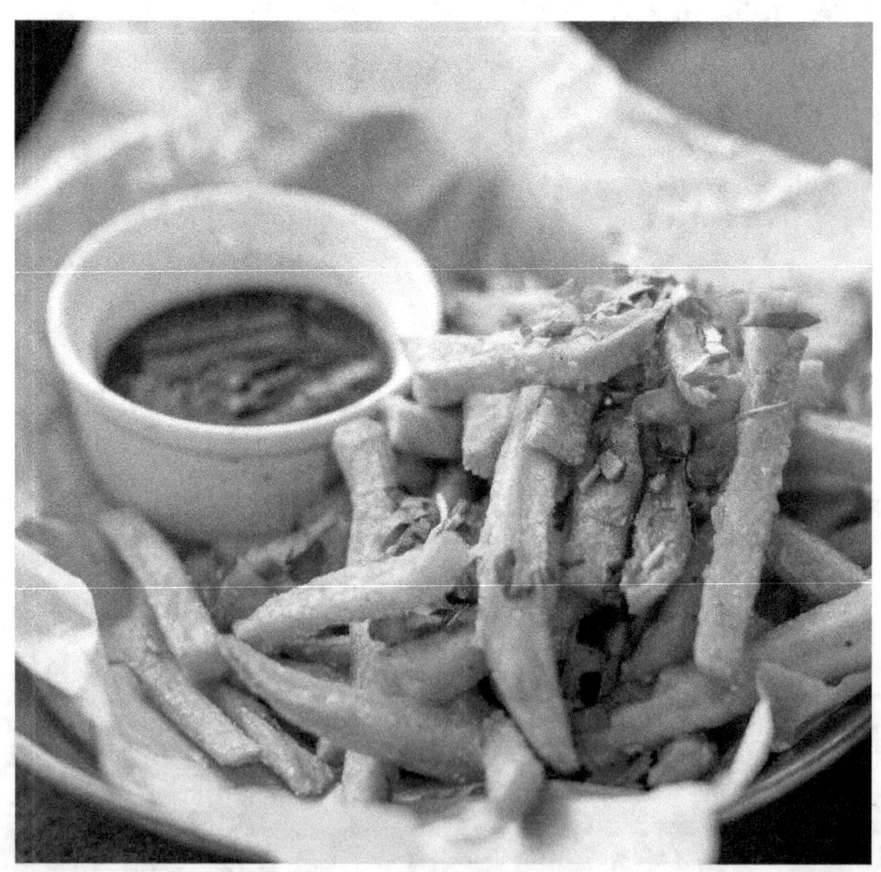

GREEK YOGURT WITH BERRIES AND ALMONDS

INGREDIENTS

- ❖ Greek yogurt (1/2 cup)
- ❖ Mixed berries (1/4 cup)
- ❖ Almonds (2 tbsp, sliced)
- ❖ Honey or maple syrup (optional, for sweetness)

INSTUCTIONS

1. In a small bowl, layer Greek yogurt, mixed berries, and sliced almonds.
2. Drizzle with honey or maple syrup if desired.
3. Enjoy this protein-rich and satisfying snack.

AVOCADO AND TOMATO RICE CAKES

INGREDIENTS

- ❖ Rice cakes (2)
- ❖ Avocado (1/2, mashed)
- ❖ Tomato (1/2, sliced)
- ❖ Sea salt and black pepper to taste

INSTUCTIONS

1. Spread mashed avocado evenly on rice cakes.
2. Top with sliced tomatoes.
3. Season with sea salt and black pepper.
4. Serve as a quick and nutritious snack.

HUMMUS WITH VEGGIE STICKS

INGREDIENTS

- ❖ Hummus (1/4 cup)
- ❖ Carrot sticks (1/2 cup)
- ❖ Cucumber sticks (1/2 cup)
- ❖ Bell pepper strips (1/2 cup)

INSTUCTIONS

1. Place hummus in a small bowl for dipping.
2. Arrange carrot sticks, cucumber sticks, and bell pepper strips on a plate.
3. Dip the vegetable sticks into hummus and enjoy this crunchy and fiber-rich snack.

HARD-BOILED EGGS WITH GUACAMOLE

INGREDIENTS

- ❖ Hard-boiled eggs (2)
- ❖ Avocado (1/2, mashed)
- ❖ Lime juice (1 tbsp)
- ❖ Cilantro (1 tbsp, chopped)
- ❖ Salt and pepper to taste

INSTUCTIONS

1. Peel and slice hard-boiled eggs in half.
2. In a bowl, mash avocado and mix with lime juice, chopped cilantro, salt, and pepper to make guacamole.
3. Top each egg half with a spoonful of guacamole.
4. Serve as a protein-packed snack option.

CHIA SEED PUDDING WITH BERRIES

INGREDIENTS

- ❖ Chia seeds (2 tbsp)
- ❖ Almond milk (1/2 cup)
- ❖ Mixed berries (1/4 cup)
- ❖ Honey or maple syrup (optional, for sweetness)

INSTUCTIONS

1. In a small jar or bowl, mix chia seeds and almond milk.
2. Let the mixture sit for 1015 minutes until thickened.
3. Top with mixed berries.
4. Sweeten with honey or maple syrup if desired.
5. Enjoy this fiber-rich and antioxidant-packed snack.

COTTAGE CHEESE AND PINEAPPLE SPEARS

INGREDIENTS

- ❖ Cottage Cheese and Pineapple Spears

INSTUCTIONS

1. Place cottage cheese in a small bowl.
2. Serve with pineapple spears for a protein-rich and refreshing snack.

TURKEY AND CHEESE ROLL-UPS

INGREDIENTS

- ❖ Turkey slices (4)
- ❖ Cheese slices (4)

INSTUCTIONS

1. Lay turkey slices flat on a cutting board.
2. Place cheese slices on top of turkey slices.
3. Roll up each turkey slice with cheese inside.
4. Secure with toothpicks if necessary.
5. Enjoy these protein-packed roll-ups as a satisfying snack.

TRAIL MIX WITH NUTS AND DRIED FRUIT

INGREDIENTS

- ❖ Almonds (1/4 cup)
- ❖ Walnuts (1/4 cup)
- ❖ Cashews (1/4 cup)
- ❖ Dried cranberries (2 tbsp)
- ❖ Dried apricots (2 tbsp, chopped)

INSTUCTIONS

1. In a bowl, mix almonds, walnuts, cashews, dried cranberries, and chopped dried apricots.
2. Portion into individual servings for a convenient and nutritious snack option.

APPLE SLICES WITH ALMOND BUTTER

INGREDIENTS

- ❖ Apple (1, sliced)
- ❖ Almond butter (2 tbsp)

INSTUCTIONS

1. Spread almond butter on apple slices.
2. Enjoy this fiber-rich and protein-packed snack for a quick energy boost.

GREEK YOGURT BARK WITH BERRIES AND ALMONDS

INGREDIENTS

* ❖ Greek yogurt (1 cup)
* ❖ Mixed berries (1/4 cup)
* ❖ Almonds (2 tbsp, sliced)
* ❖ Honey or maple syrup (optional, for sweetness)

INSTUCTIONS

1. Line a baking sheet with parchment paper.
2. Spread Greek yogurt evenly on the parchment paper.
3. Sprinkle mixed berries and sliced almonds over the yogurt.
4. Drizzle with honey or maple syrup if desired.
5. Freeze for 23 hours until firm.
6. Break into pieces and enjoy this frozen treat as a healthy snack option.

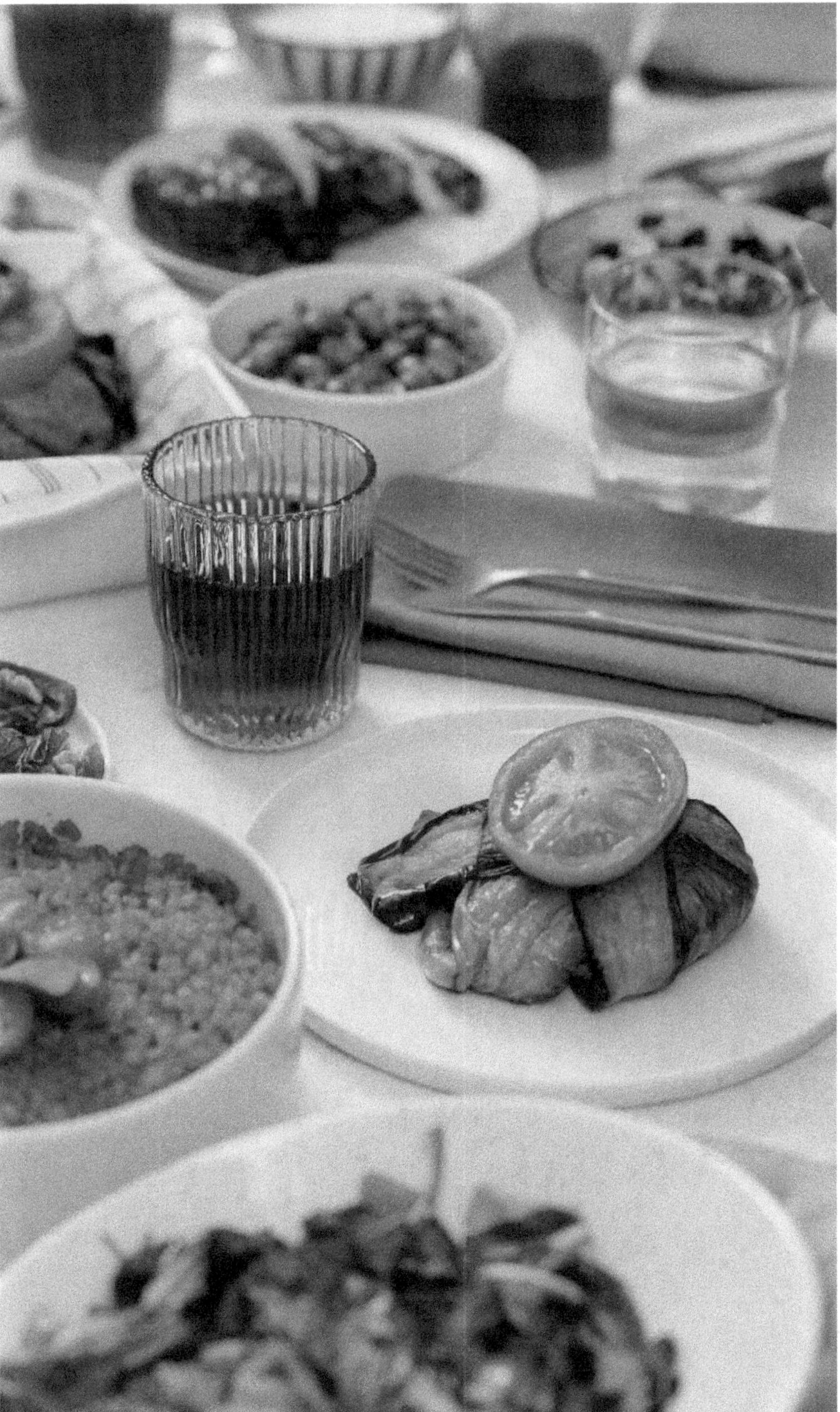

Fish and Seafood

recipes

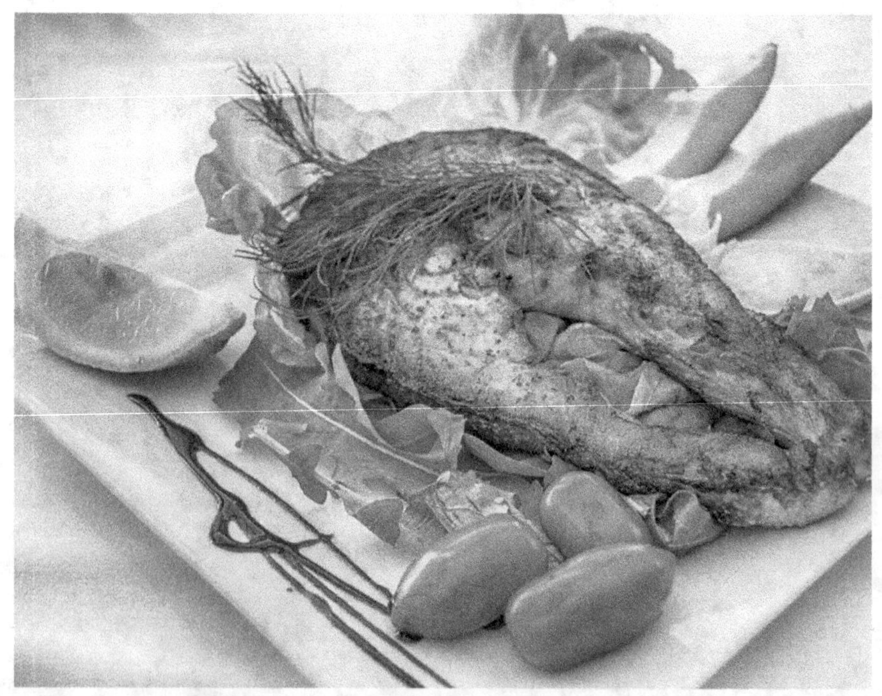

GRILLED SALMON WITH LEMON AND DILL

INGREDIENTS

- ❖ Salmon fillets (2)
- ❖ Lemon (1, sliced)
- ❖ Fresh dill (2 tbsp, chopped)
- ❖ Olive oil (2 tbsp)
- ❖ Salt and pepper to taste

INSTUCTIONS

1. Preheat the grill to medium-high heat.
2. Rub salmon fillets with olive oil and season with salt, pepper, and chopped dill.
3. Place lemon slices on top of each salmon fillet.
4. Grill salmon for 45 minutes on each side or until cooked through.
5. Serve hot with additional lemon wedges if desired.

BAKED COD WITH TOMATO AND BASIL

INGREDIENTS

- ❖ Cod fillets (2)
- ❖ Tomato (1, sliced)
- ❖ Fresh basil leaves (1/4 cup)
- ❖ Garlic (1 clove, minced)
- ❖ Olive oil (2 tbsp)
- ❖ Salt and pepper to taste

INSTUCTIONS

1. Preheat the oven to 375°F (190°C).
2. Place cod fillets on a baking dish lined with parchment paper.
3. Drizzle olive oil over cod fillets and sprinkle minced garlic on top.
4. Arrange tomato slices and fresh basil leaves on top of the cod.
5. Season with salt and pepper.
6. Bake for 1520 minutes or until fish is cooked through and flakes easily with a fork.
7. Serve hot and enjoy this flavorful dish.

SHRIMP STIR-FRY WITH VEGETABLES

INGREDIENTS

- Shrimp (1/2 lb, peeled and deveined)
- Broccoli florets (1 cup)
- Bell peppers (1/2 cup, sliced)
- Carrots (1/2 cup, sliced)
- Snow peas (1/2 cup)
- Garlic (2 cloves, minced)
- Ginger (1 tsp, grated)
- Soy sauce (2 tbsp)
- Sesame oil (1 tbsp)
- Olive oil (1 tbsp)

INSTUCTIONS

1. Heat olive oil in a skillet or wok over medium-high heat.
2. Add minced garlic and grated ginger to the skillet and cook until fragrant.
3. Add shrimp to the skillet and cook until pink and opaque.
4. Stir in broccoli florets, sliced bell peppers, carrots, and snow peas.
5. Cook until vegetables are tender-crisp.
6. Add soy sauce and sesame oil to the skillet and toss to combine.
7. Serve hot and enjoy this quick and nutritious stir-fry.

TUNA SALAD WITH AVOCADO AND CHICKPEAS

INGREDIENTS

- ❖ Canned tuna (1 can, drained)
- ❖ Avocado (1, diced)
- ❖ Chickpeas (1/2 cup, drained and rinsed)
- ❖ Red onion (1/4 cup, diced)
- ❖ Celery (1/4 cup, diced)
- ❖ Lemon juice (1 tbsp)
- ❖ Olive oil (1 tbsp)
- ❖ Fresh parsley (2 tbsp, chopped)
- ❖ Salt and pepper to taste

INSTUCTIONS

1. In a bowl, combine canned tuna, diced avocado, chickpeas, diced red onion, diced celery, chopped parsley, lemon juice, and olive oil.
2. Season with salt and pepper to taste.
3. Mix until well combined.
4. Serve chilled as a delicious and protein-packed salad.

SALMON AND ASPARAGUS FOIL PACKETS

INGREDIENTS

- ❖ Salmon fillets (2)
- ❖ Asparagus spears (1 bunch)
- ❖ Lemon (1, sliced)
- ❖ Garlic (2 cloves, minced)
- ❖ Olive oil (2 tbsp)
- ❖ Salt and pepper to taste

INSTUCTIONS

1. Preheat the oven to 375°F (190°C).
2. Place salmon fillets on pieces of aluminum foil.
3. Arrange asparagus spears around the salmon.
4. Drizzle olive oil over the salmon and asparagus.
5. Sprinkle minced garlic on top.
6. Season with salt and pepper.
7. Place lemon slices on top of each salmon fillet.
8. Seal the foil packets tightly.
9. Bake for 2025 minutes or until salmon is cooked through and asparagus is tender.
10. Serve hot and enjoy this easy and flavorful dish.

SEARED SCALLOPS WITH SPINACH AND GARLIC BUTTER

INGREDIENTS

- ❖ Scallops (1/2 lb)
- ❖ Baby spinach (2 cups)
- ❖ Garlic (2 cloves, minced)
- ❖ Butter (2 tbsp)
- ❖ Olive oil (1 tbsp)
- ❖ Lemon juice (1 tbsp)
- ❖ Salt and pepper to taste

INSTUCTIONS

1. Pat dry scallops with paper towels and season with salt and pepper.
2. Heat olive oil in a skillet over medium-high heat.
3. Add scallops to the skillet and cook for 23 minutes on each side until golden brown and opaque.
4. Remove scallops from the skillet and set aside.
5. In the same skillet, melt butter and add minced garlic.
6. Add baby spinach to the skillet and cook until wilted.
7. Stir in lemon juice and season with salt and pepper.
8. Return scallops to the skillet briefly to reheat.
9. Serve hot and enjoy this elegant and flavorful dish.

BAKED HALIBUT WITH HERBED QUINOA

INGREDIENTS

- ❖ Halibut fillets (2)
- ❖ Quinoa (1 cup, cooked)
- ❖ Fresh herbs (such as parsley, dill, and chives) (1/4 cup, chopped)
- ❖ Lemon zest (1 tsp)
- ❖ Garlic (1 clove, minced)
- ❖ Olive oil (2 tbsp)
- ❖ Salt and pepper to taste

INSTUCTIONS

1. Preheat the oven to 375°F (190°C).
2. Season halibut fillets with salt, pepper, minced garlic, and lemon zest.
3. Drizzle olive oil over halibut fillets.
4. Place halibut fillets on a baking dish lined with parchment paper.
5. Bake for 1520 minutes or until fish is cooked through and flakes easily with a fork.
6. In a bowl, mix cooked quinoa with chopped fresh herbs.
7. Serve baked halibut over herbed quinoa.
8. Enjoy this light and nutritious seafood dish.

TUNA LETTUCE WRAPS WITH CUCUMBER AND AVOCADO

INGREDIENTS

- Canned tuna (1 can, drained)
- Avocado (1/2, diced)
- Cucumber (1/2, sliced)
- Lettuce leaves (4)
- Red onion (1/4 cup, diced)
- Dijon mustard (1 tbsp)
- Olive oil (1 tbsp)
- Lemon juice (1 tbsp)
- Salt and pepper to taste

INSTUCTIONS

1. In a bowl, combine canned tuna, diced avocado, diced red onion, Dijon mustard, olive oil, lemon juice, salt, and pepper.
2. Mix until well combined.
3. Lay lettuce leaves flat on a plate.
4. Spoon tuna mixture onto lettuce leaves.
5. Top with sliced cucumber.
6. Roll up lettuce leaves to form wraps.
7. Serve immediately and enjoy this low-carb and protein-rich snack.

SHRIMP AND VEGETABLE SKEWERS

INGREDIENTS

- Shrimp (1/2 lb, peeled and deveined)
- Cherry tomatoes (1 cup)
- Bell peppers (1/2 cup, diced)
- Zucchini (1/2 cup, sliced)
- Red onion (1/4 cup, diced)
- Olive oil (2 tbsp)
- Garlic (2 cloves, minced)
- Lemon juice (1 tbsp)
- Salt and pepper to taste

INSTUCTIONS

1. In a bowl, combine peeled and deveined shrimp with diced bell peppers, sliced zucchini, diced red onion, minced garlic, olive oil, lemon juice, salt, and pepper.
2. Toss until shrimp and vegetables are evenly coated.
3. Thread shrimp and vegetables onto skewers.
4. Preheat a grill or grill pan over medium-high heat.
5. Grill skewers for 23 minutes on each side or until shrimp are pink and opaque.
6. Serve hot and enjoy these flavorful shrimp and vegetable skewers.

SALMON SALAD WITH LEMON DILL DRESSING

INGREDIENTS

- Salmon fillets (2)
- Mixed salad greens (4 cups)
- Cherry tomatoes (1 cup, halved)
- Cucumber (1/2, sliced)
- Red onion (1/4 cup, thinly sliced)
- Fresh dill (2 tbsp, chopped)
- Lemon juice (2 tbsp)
- Olive oil (2 tbsp)

INSTUCTIONS

1. Season salmon fillets with salt and pepper.
2. Heat olive oil in a skillet over medium-high heat.
3. Add salmon fillets to the skillet and cook for 34 minutes on each side until cooked through.
4. Remove salmon from the skillet and let cool slightly.
5. In a small bowl, whisk together lemon juice, olive oil, chopped dill, salt, and pepper to make the dressing.
6. In a large bowl, combine mixed salad greens, halved cherry tomatoes, sliced cucumber, and thinly sliced red onion.
7. Flake cooked salmon into bite-sized pieces and add to the salad.
8. Drizzle salad with lemon dill dressing and toss until well coated.

9. Serve immediately and enjoy this light and refreshing
   salad with salmon.

Poultry and Meats

recipes

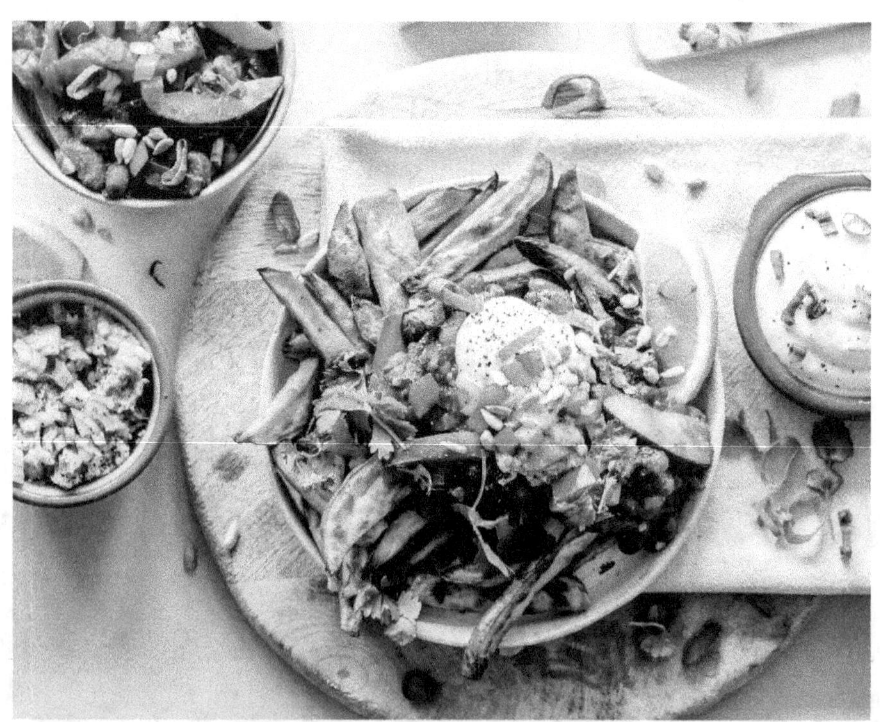

GRILLED CHICKEN WITH HERBED QUINOA SALAD

INGREDIENTS

- ❖ Chicken breasts (2)
- ❖ Quinoa (1 cup, cooked)
- ❖ Cherry tomatoes (1 cup, halved)
- ❖ Cucumber (1/2, diced)
- ❖ Red onion (1/4 cup, thinly sliced)
- ❖ Fresh parsley (2 tbsp, chopped)
- ❖ Fresh mint (2 tbsp, chopped)
- ❖ Olive oil (2 tbsp)
- ❖ Lemon juice (2 tbsp)
- ❖ Salt and pepper to taste

INSTUCTIONS

1. Preheat the grill to medium-high heat.
2. Season chicken breasts with salt, pepper, and olive oil.
3. Grill chicken for 68 minutes on each side or until cooked through.
4. In a large bowl, combine cooked quinoa, halved cherry tomatoes, diced cucumber, thinly sliced red onion, chopped parsley, chopped mint, olive oil, lemon juice, salt, and pepper.
5. Toss until well combined.
6. Serve grilled chicken over herbed quinoa salad.
7. Enjoy this protein-rich and flavorful dish

TURKEY MEATBALLS WITH ZUCCHINI NOODLES

INGREDIENTS

- Ground turkey (1 lb)
- Onion (1/2, finely chopped)
- Garlic (2 cloves, minced)
- Almond flour (1/4 cup)
- Fresh parsley (2 tbsp, chopped)
- Egg (1)
- Salt and pepper to taste
- Zucchini (2, spiralized into noodles)
- Olive oil (2 tbsp)
- Tomato sauce (1 cup)

INSTUCTIONS

1. Preheat the oven to 375°F (190°C).
2. In a bowl, combine ground turkey, finely chopped onion, minced garlic, almond flour, egg, chopped parsley, salt, and pepper.
3. Roll the mixture into meatballs and place them on a baking sheet lined with parchment paper.
4. Bake meatballs for 2025 minutes or until cooked through.
5. In a skillet, heat olive oil over medium heat.
6. Add spiralized zucchini noodles to the skillet and cook until tender.
7. Heat tomato sauce in a separate saucepan.
8. Serve turkey meatballs over zucchini noodles with warm tomato sauce.
9. Enjoy this low-carb and nutritious meal.

BEEF STIR-FRY WITH BROCCOLI AND BELL PEPPERS

INGREDIENTS

- Beef sirloin or flank steak (1 lb, thinly sliced)
- Broccoli florets (2 cups)
- Bell peppers (1, sliced)
- Onion (1, sliced)
- Garlic (2 cloves, minced)
- Soy sauce (3 tbsp)
- Sesame oil (1 tbsp)
- Olive oil (2 tbsp)
- Ginger (1 tsp, grated)
- Salt and pepper to taste

INSTUCTIONS

1. In a bowl, marinate thinly sliced beef with minced garlic, soy sauce, sesame oil, grated ginger, salt, and pepper for 1530 minutes.
2. Heat olive oil in a skillet or wok over medium-high heat.
3. Add marinated beef slices to the skillet and cook until browned.
4. Remove beef from the skillet and set aside.
5. In the same skillet, add sliced onion, broccoli florets, and sliced bell peppers.
6. Stir-fry vegetables until tender-crisp.
7. Return cooked beef to the skillet and toss to combine with vegetables.
8. Serve hot and enjoy this flavorful beef stir-fry.

BAKED CHICKEN THIGHS WITH SWEET POTATO MASH

INGREDIENTS

- Chicken thighs (4)
- Sweet potatoes (2, peeled and diced)
- Olive oil (2 tbsp)
- Garlic powder (1 tsp)
- Paprika (1 tsp)
- Salt and pepper to taste
- Fresh parsley (2 tbsp, chopped)

INSTUCTIONS

1. Preheat the oven to 400°F (200°C).
2. Season chicken thighs with olive oil, garlic powder, paprika, salt, and pepper.
3. Place chicken thighs on a baking sheet lined with parchment paper.
4. Bake chicken thighs for 2530 minutes or until cooked through and juices run clear.
5. Meanwhile, boil diced sweet potatoes in water until tender.
6. Drain cooked sweet potatoes and mash with a fork.
7. Season sweet potato mash with salt, pepper, and chopped parsley.
8. Serve baked chicken thighs with sweet potato mash.
9. Enjoy this comforting and nutritious meal.

TURKEY AND VEGETABLE SKEWERS WITH TZATZIKI

INGREDIENTS

- Ground turkey (1 lb)
- Zucchini (2, sliced)
- Cherry tomatoes (1 cup)
- Red onion (1, sliced)
- Olive oil (2 tbsp)
- Lemon juice (2 tbsp)
- Garlic (2 cloves, minced)
- Fresh oregano (1 tbsp, chopped)
- Salt and pepper to taste
- Wooden skewers
- Tzatziki sauce (for serving)

INSTUCTIONS

1. Soak wooden skewers in water for at least 30 minutes to prevent burning.
2. In a bowl, combine ground turkey with minced garlic, chopped oregano, olive oil, lemon juice, salt, and pepper.
3. Mix until well combined.
4. Thread ground turkey, sliced zucchini, cherry tomatoes, and sliced red onion onto skewers.
5. Preheat a grill or grill pan over medium-high heat.
6. Grill skewers for 68 minutes on each side or until turkey is cooked through and vegetables are tender.
7. Serve hot with tzatziki sauce for dipping.
8. Enjoy these flavorful turkey and vegetable skewers.

PORK TENDERLOIN WITH APPLE AND SAGE SAUCE

INGREDIENTS

- Pork tenderloin (1 lb)
- Apples (2, peeled and diced)
- Fresh sage leaves (8)
- Garlic (2 cloves, minced)
- Chicken broth (1/2 cup)
- Olive oil (2 tbsp)
- Salt and pepper to taste

INSTUCTIONS

1. Preheat the oven to 375°F (190°C).
2. Season pork tenderloin with salt and pepper.
3. Heat olive oil in an oven-safe skillet over medium-high heat.
4. Sear pork tenderloin on all sides until browned.
5. Remove pork tenderloin from the skillet and set aside.
6. In the same skillet, add diced apples, minced garlic, and fresh sage leaves.
7. Cook until apples are softened and fragrant.
8. Return pork tenderloin to the skillet and pour chicken broth over the top.
9. Transfer the skillet to the oven and bake for 1520 minutes or until pork is cooked through.
10. Serve hot with apple and sage sauce drizzled over the top.
11. Enjoy this delicious and savory pork tenderloin dish.

CHICKEN CURRY WITH CAULIFLOWER RICE

INGREDIENTS

- ❖ Chicken breast (2, diced)
- ❖ Cauliflower (1, grated into rice-like texture)
- ❖ Onion (1, diced)
- ❖ Garlic (2 cloves, minced)
- ❖ Ginger (1 tsp, grated)
- ❖ Coconut milk (1 can)
- ❖ Curry powder (2 tbsp)
- ❖ Turmeric powder (1 tsp)
- ❖ Cumin powder (1 tsp)
- ❖ Olive oil (2 tbsp)
- ❖ Salt and pepper to taste

INSTUCTIONS

1. Heat olive oil in a skillet over medium heat.
2. Add diced chicken breast to the skillet and cook until browned.
3. Remove chicken from the skillet and set aside.
4. In the same skillet, add diced onion, minced garlic, and grated ginger.
5. Cook until onion is softened and fragrant.
6. Add grated cauliflower to the skillet and cook until tender.
7. Stir in curry powder, turmeric powder, and cumin powder.
8. Pour coconut milk into the skillet and bring to a simmer.
9. Return cooked chicken to the skillet and simmer for 1015 minutes.
10. Season with salt and pepper to taste.

11. Serve hot with cauliflower rice.
12. Enjoy this flavorful and satisfying chicken curry dish.

BEEF AND VEGETABLE STIR-FRY
WITH BROWN RICE

INGREDIENTS

- ❖ Beef sirloin or flank steak (1 lb, thinly sliced)
- ❖ Broccoli florets (2 cups)
- ❖ Carrots (2, sliced)
- ❖ Bell peppers (1, sliced)
- ❖ Onion (1, sliced)
- ❖ Garlic (2 cloves, minced)
- ❖ Soy sauce (3 tbsp)
- ❖ Olive oil (2 tbsp)
- ❖ Brown rice (2 cups, cooked)
- ❖ Salt and pepper to taste

INSTUCTIONS

1. Heat olive oil in a skillet or wok over medium-high heat.
2. Add thinly sliced beef to the skillet and cook until browned.
3. Remove beef from the skillet and set aside.
4. In the same skillet, add minced garlic, sliced onion, sliced carrots, sliced bell peppers, and broccoli florets.
5. Stir-fry vegetables until tender-crisp.
6. Return cooked beef to the skillet and toss to combine with vegetables.
7. Add soy sauce to the skillet and stir until everything is well coated.
8. Serve hot with cooked brown rice.
9. Enjoy this hearty and nutritious beef stir-fry.

LEMON HERB ROAST CHICKEN WITH ROASTED VEGETABLES

INGREDIENTS

- Whole chicken (1, about 4 lbs)
- Potatoes (4, peeled and quartered)
- Carrots (4, peeled and chopped)
- Onion (1, quartered)
- Garlic (4 cloves, minced)
- Lemon (1, sliced)
- Fresh rosemary (2 sprigs)
- Fresh thyme (4 sprigs)
- Olive oil (3 tbsp)
- Salt and pepper to taste

INSTUCTIONS

1. Preheat the oven to 425°F (220°C).
2. Rinse the whole chicken and pat dry with paper towels.
3. Season the chicken generously with salt and pepper, inside and out.
4. Stuff the cavity of the chicken with minced garlic, lemon slices, fresh rosemary, and fresh thyme.
5. Tie the legs together with kitchen twine.
6. Place quartered potatoes, chopped carrots, quartered onion, and remaining garlic cloves in a roasting pan.
7. Drizzle olive oil over the vegetables and season with salt and pepper.
8. Place the seasoned chicken on top of the vegetables in the roasting pan.
9. Roast in the preheated oven for 15 minutes, then reduce the temperature to 375°F (190°C) and continue roasting

for about 1 hour and 15 minutes, or until the internal temperature of the chicken reaches 165°F (74°C) and the juices run clear.

10. Remove the chicken from the oven and let it rest for about 10 minutes before carving.
11. Serve the roast chicken with roasted vegetables.
12. Enjoy this classic and comforting roast chicken dinner.

SPICY TURKEY CHILI WITH BEANS

INGREDIENTS

- Ground turkey (1 lb)
- Onion (1, diced)
- Bell peppers (2, diced)
- Garlic (4 cloves, minced)
- Tomato paste (1 can)
- Diced tomatoes (1 can)
- Black beans (1 can, drained and rinsed)
- Kidney beans (1 can, drained and rinsed)
- Chili powder (2 tbsp)
- Cumin powder (1 tbsp)
- Paprika (1 tbsp)
- Cayenne pepper (1/2 tsp, optional)
- Olive oil (2 tbsp)
- Salt and pepper to taste

INSTUCTIONS

1. In a bowl, mix chia seeds and coconut milk.
2. Let the mixture sit for 1015 minutes until thickened.
3. Stir in diced mango and shredded coconut.
4. Sweeten with honey or maple syrup if desired.
5. Divide the chia seed pudding into serving cups and refrigerate for at least 1 hour.
6. Serve chilled and enjoy this refreshing breakfast.

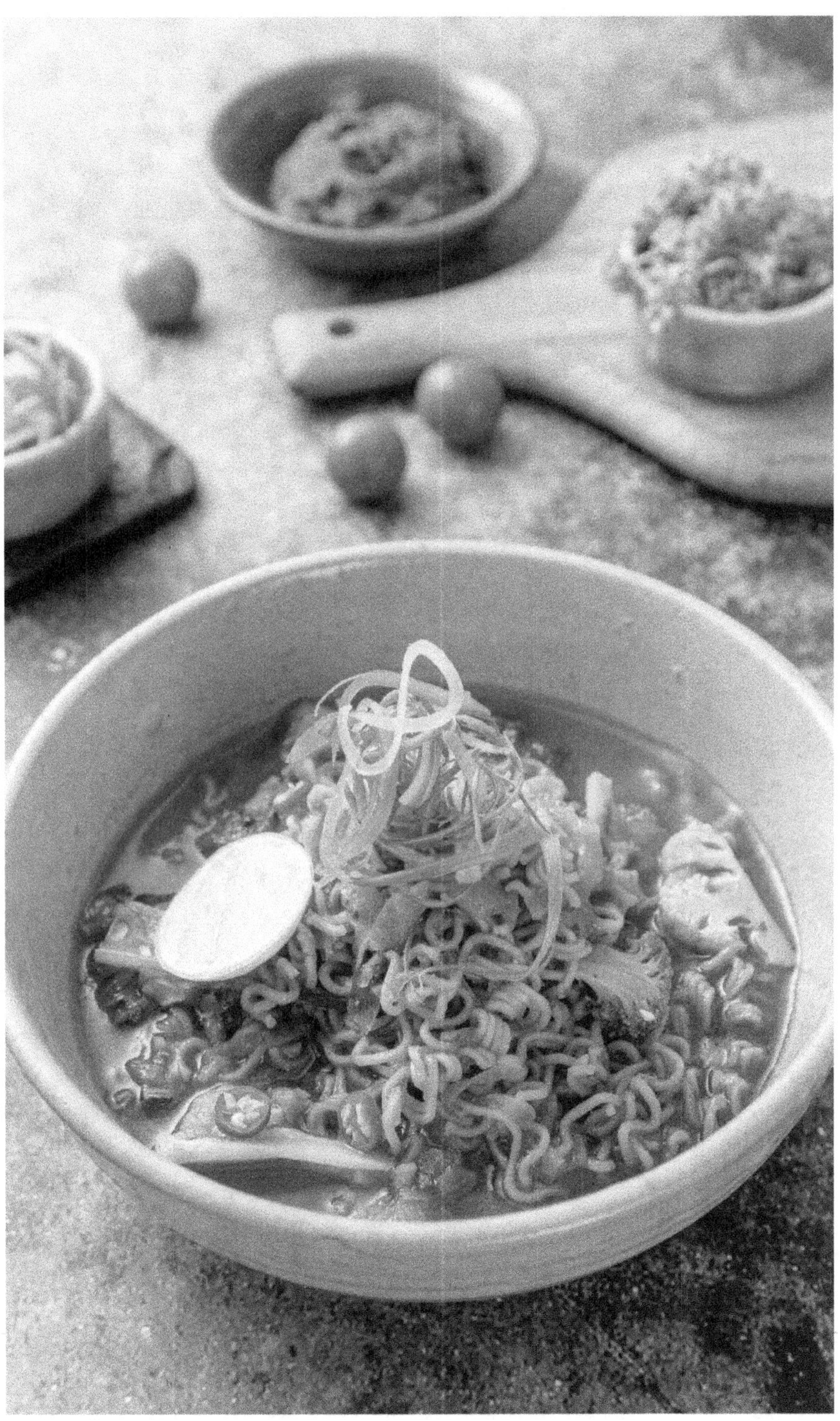

Gluten-Free

recipes

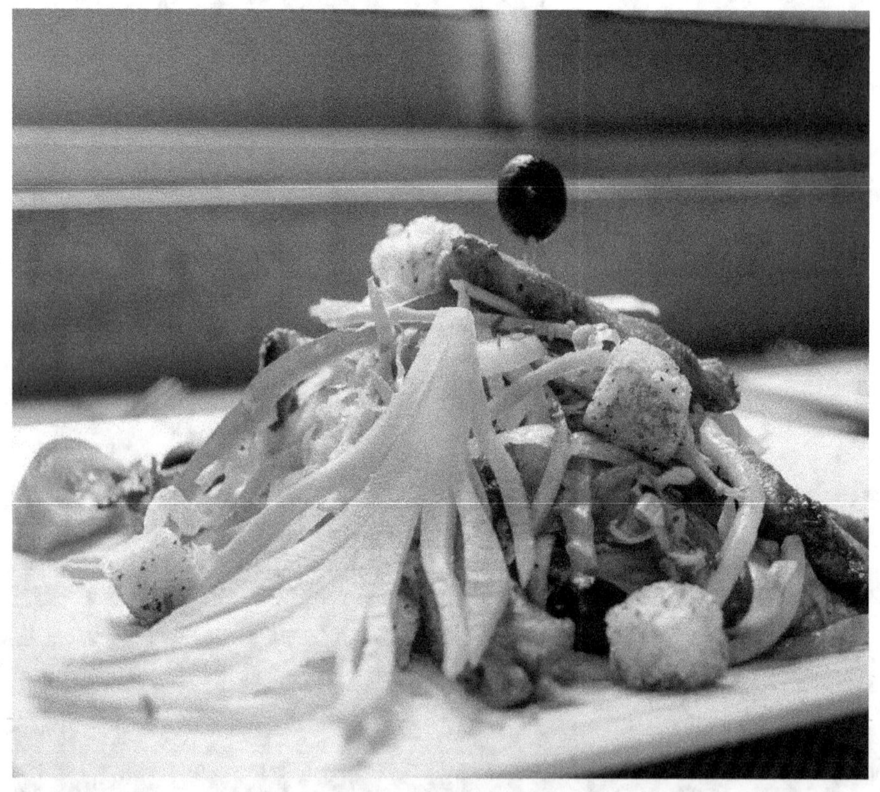

QUINOA-STUFFED BELL PEPPERS

INGREDIENTS

- ❖ Bell peppers (4, halved and seeds removed)
- ❖ Quinoa (1 cup, cooked)
- ❖ Ground turkey or beef (1/2 lb, cooked)
- ❖ Onion (1, diced)
- ❖ Garlic (2 cloves, minced)
- ❖ Tomato sauce (1 cup)
- ❖ Italian seasoning (1 tsp)
- ❖ Salt and pepper to taste
- ❖ Olive oil (2 tbsp)
- ❖ Shredded cheese (optional, for topping)

INSTUCTIONS

1. Preheat the oven to 375°F (190°C).
2. Heat olive oil in a skillet over medium heat.
3. Add diced onion and minced garlic to the skillet and cook until softened.
4. Add cooked ground turkey or beef to the skillet and season with Italian seasoning, salt, and pepper. Cook until browned.
5. Stir in cooked quinoa and tomato sauce, and cook for a few more minutes.
6. Place halved bell peppers in a baking dish.
7. Spoon the quinoa and meat mixture into each bell pepper half.
8. If desired, top each stuffed pepper with shredded cheese.
9. Cover the baking dish with foil and bake for 25-30 minutes, until the peppers are tender.
10. Serve hot and enjoy this flavorful and nutritious dish.

ZUCCHINI NOODLES WITH PESTO AND CHERRY TOMATOES

INGREDIENTS

- Zucchini (2, spiralized into noodles)
- Cherry tomatoes (1 cup, halved)
- Basil pesto (1/2 cup)
- Garlic (2 cloves, minced)
- Olive oil (2 tbsp)
- Salt and pepper to taste
- Grated Parmesan cheese (optional, for topping)

INSTUCTIONS

1. Heat olive oil in a skillet over medium heat.
2. Add minced garlic to the skillet and cook until fragrant.
3. Add zucchini noodles to the skillet and cook for 23 minutes, until tender.
4. Stir in cherry tomatoes and cook for an additional 12 minutes.
5. Remove the skillet from heat and add basil pesto to the zucchini noodles and cherry tomatoes. Toss until evenly coated.
6. Season with salt and pepper to taste.
7. If desired, top with grated Parmesan cheese before serving.
8. Serve hot and enjoy this light and flavorful gluten-free meal.

GRILLED LEMON HERB CHICKEN WITH ROASTED

INGREDIENTS

- ❖ Chicken breasts (2)
- ❖ Lemon (1, juiced)
- ❖ Olive oil (2 tbsp)
- ❖ Fresh herbs (such as rosemary, thyme, and parsley) (2 tbsp, chopped)
- ❖ Garlic (2 cloves, minced)
- ❖ Salt and pepper to taste
- ❖ Assorted vegetables (such as bell peppers, zucchini, and carrots) (4 cups, chopped)
- ❖ Olive oil (2 tbsp)
- ❖ Salt and pepper to taste

INSTUCTIONS

1. In a bowl, mix together lemon juice, olive oil, chopped herbs, minced garlic, salt, and pepper.
2. Add chicken breasts to the bowl and marinate for at least 30 minutes.
3. Preheat the grill to medium-high heat.
4. Grill chicken breasts for 68 minutes on each side, until cooked through and juices run clear.
5. While the chicken is grilling, preheat the oven to 400°F (200°C).
6. Toss chopped vegetables with olive oil, salt, and pepper on a baking sheet.
7. Roast vegetables in the preheated oven for 2530 minutes, until tender and lightly browned.

8. Serve grilled lemon herb chicken with roasted vegetables.
9. Enjoy this delicious and healthy gluten-free meal.

SALMON AND AVOCADO SALAD WITH CITRUS DRESSING

INGREDIENTS

- Salmon fillets (2)
- Mixed salad greens (4 cups)
- Avocado (1, diced)
- Cherry tomatoes (1 cup, halved)
- Red onion (1/4 cup, thinly sliced)
- Olive oil (2 tbsp)
- Lemon juice (2 tbsp)
- Orange juice (2 tbsp)
- Dijon mustard (1 tsp)
- Honey (1 tsp)
- Salt and pepper to taste

INSTUCTIONS

1. Season salmon fillets with salt and pepper.
2. Heat olive oil in a skillet over medium-high heat.
3. Add salmon fillets to the skillet and cook for 45 minutes on each side, until cooked through.
4. In a small bowl, whisk together lemon juice, orange juice, Dijon mustard, honey, salt, and pepper to make the dressing.
5. In a large bowl, toss mixed salad greens, diced avocado, halved cherry tomatoes, and thinly sliced red onion with the citrus dressing.
6. Divide salad onto plates and top each with a cooked salmon fillet.

7. Serve immediately and enjoy this fresh and vibrant gluten-free salad.

STUFFED SWEET POTATOES WITH BLACK BEANS AND

INGREDIENTS

- Sweet potatoes (2)
- Black beans (1 can, drained and rinsed)
- Avocado (1, diced)
- Red onion (1/4 cup, diced)
- Cilantro (2 tbsp, chopped)
- Lime (1, juiced)
- Olive oil (1 tbsp)
- Salt and pepper to taste

INSTUCTIONS

1. Preheat the oven to 400°F (200°C).
2. Pierce sweet potatoes with a fork and place them on a baking sheet lined with parchment paper.
3. Bake sweet potatoes for 4555 minutes, until tender.
4. In a bowl, mix together black beans, diced avocado, diced red onion, chopped cilantro, lime juice, olive oil, salt, and pepper.
5. Once sweet potatoes are cooked, slice them open lengthwise and fluff the insides with a fork.
6. Spoon the black bean and avocado mixture into each sweet potato.
7. Serve hot and enjoy these flavorful and satisfying stuffed sweet potatoes.

Dairy-Free
recipes

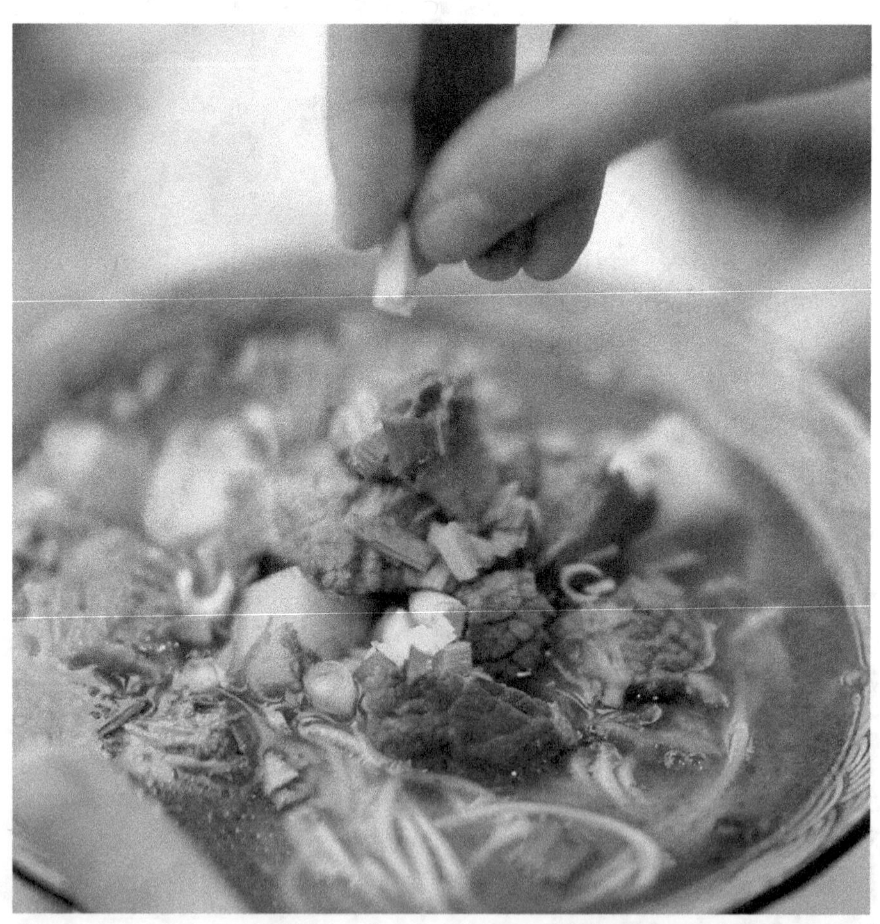

COCONUT CURRY LENTIL SOUP

INGREDIENTS

- Red lentils (1 cup)
- Coconut milk (1 can)
- Vegetable broth (4 cups)
- Onion (1, diced)
- Celery stalk (1, diced)
- Garlic (2 cloves, minced)
- Ginger (1-inch piece, grated)
- Carrot (1, diced)
- Curry powder (2 tbsp)
- Turmeric powder (1 tsp)
- Cumin powder (1 tsp)
- Olive oil (2 tbsp)
- Salt and pepper to taste
- Fresh cilantro (for garnish)

INSTUCTIONS

1. Heat olive oil in a large pot over medium heat.
2. Add diced onion, carrot, and celery to the pot and sauté until softened.
3. Stir in minced garlic and grated ginger, and cook for another minute.
4. Add curry powder, turmeric powder, and cumin powder to the pot, and stir to combine with the vegetables.
5. Pour in vegetable broth and bring to a boil.
6. Add red lentils to the pot and reduce heat to simmer. Cook for about 1520 minutes, until lentils are tender.
7. Stir in coconut milk and season with salt and pepper to taste.
8. Continue to simmer for another 510 minutes to allow flavors to meld.

9. Serve hot, garnished with fresh cilantro.
10. Enjoy this creamy and flavorful dairy-free soup.

GRILLED LEMON HERB SHRIMP SKEWERS

INGREDIENTS

- ❖ Shrimp (1 lb, peeled and deveined)
- ❖ Lemon (1, juiced)
- ❖ Olive oil (2 tbsp)
- ❖ Fresh parsley (2 tbsp, chopped)
- ❖ Fresh dill (2 tbsp, chopped)
- ❖ Garlic (2 cloves, minced)
- ❖ Salt and pepper to taste
- ❖ Wooden skewers

INSTUCTIONS

1. In a bowl, combine lemon juice, olive oil, chopped parsley, chopped dill, minced garlic, salt, and pepper.
2. Add peeled and deveined shrimp to the bowl and toss to coat evenly.
3. Cover and marinate in the refrigerator for at least 30 minutes.
4. Preheat the grill to medium-high heat.
5. Thread marinated shrimp onto wooden skewers.
6. Grill shrimp skewers for 23 minutes on each side, until shrimp are pink and opaque.
7. Serve hot and enjoy these zesty and flavorful shrimp skewers.

STUFFED BELL PEPPERS WITH QUINOA AND BLACK BEANS

INGREDIENTS

- Bell peppers (4, halved and seeds removed)
- Quinoa (1 cup, cooked)
- Black beans (1 can, drained and rinsed)
- Onion (1, diced)
- Garlic (2 cloves, minced)
- Cumin powder (1 tsp)
- Chili powder (1 tsp)
- Olive oil (2 tbsp)
- Salt and pepper to taste
- Avocado (1, diced, for garnish)
- Fresh cilantro (for garnish)

INSTUCTIONS

1. Preheat the oven to 375°F (190°C).
2. Heat olive oil in a skillet over medium heat.
3. Add diced onion and minced garlic to the skillet and sauté until softened.
4. Stir in cooked quinoa, drained and rinsed black beans, cumin powder, chili powder, salt, and pepper.
5. Cook for another 23 minutes to allow flavors to meld.
6. Stuff halved bell peppers with the quinoa and black bean mixture.
7. Place stuffed bell peppers in a baking dish.
8. Cover the baking dish with foil and bake for 2530 minutes, until peppers are tender.
9. Remove from the oven and garnish with diced avocado and fresh cilantro.

10. Serve hot and enjoy these hearty and nutritious stuffed peppers.

LEMON GARLIC ROASTED VEGETABLES

INGREDIENTS

* ❖ Assorted vegetables (such as carrots, broccoli, and cauliflower) (4 cups, chopped)
* ❖ Lemon (1, juiced)
* ❖ Olive oil (2 tbsp)
* ❖ Garlic (2 cloves, minced)
* ❖ Salt and pepper to taste

INSTUCTIONS

1. Preheat the oven to 400°F (200°C).
2. In a large bowl, toss chopped vegetables with olive oil, minced garlic, lemon juice, salt, and pepper until evenly coated.
3. Spread seasoned vegetables in a single layer on a baking sheet lined with parchment paper.
4. Roast in the preheated oven for 2530 minutes, stirring halfway through, until vegetables are tender and lightly browned.
5. Remove from the oven and serve hot as a delicious and nutritious side dish.

CREAMY AVOCADO PASTA

INGREDIENTS

- ❖ Gluten-free pasta (8 oz)
- ❖ Avocado (2, peeled and pitted)
- ❖ Garlic (2 cloves, minced)
- ❖ Lemon (1, juiced)
- ❖ Olive oil (2 tbsp)
- ❖ Fresh basil leaves (1/4 cup, chopped)
- ❖ Salt and pepper to taste
- ❖ Cherry tomatoes (1 cup, halved, optional, for garnish)

INSTUCTIONS

1. In a bowl, mix chia seeds and coconut milk.
2. Let the mixture sit for 1015 minutes until thickened.
3. Stir in diced mango and shredded coconut.
4. Sweeten with honey or maple syrup if desired.
5. Divide the chia seed pudding into serving cups and refrigerate for at least 1 hour.
6. Serve chilled and enjoy this refreshing breakfast.

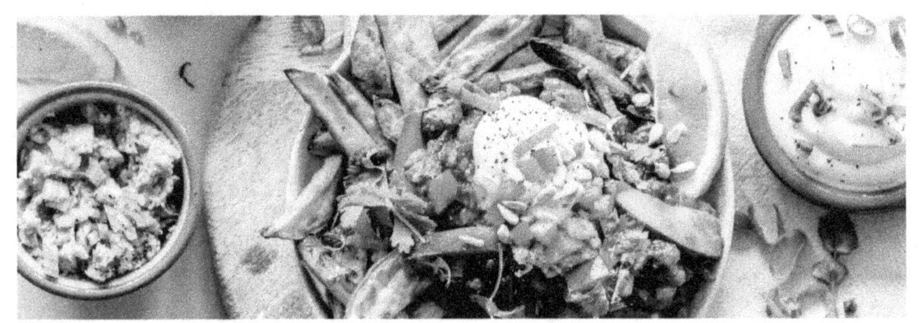

CONCLUSION

In conclusion, this Hashimoto's diet cookbook offers a comprehensive approach to managing Hashimoto's disease through nutritious and delicious meals. By focusing on whole, nutrient-dense foods and avoiding potential triggers, individuals can support their thyroid health and overall well-being.

The diverse range of recipes provides ample variety, ensuring enjoyment and satisfaction while adhering to dietary guidelines. From flavorful soups and salads to hearty mains and snacks, each recipe is thoughtfully crafted to nourish the body and soothe symptoms associated with Hashimoto's disease.

Embracing this dietary approach not only offers relief from symptoms but also empowers individuals to take control of their health journey. As you embark on this path, remember that every meal is an opportunity to fuel your body with the nourishment it needs to thrive.

With dedication and determination, adopting and adapting to this diet can pave the way to a healthier, happier you.

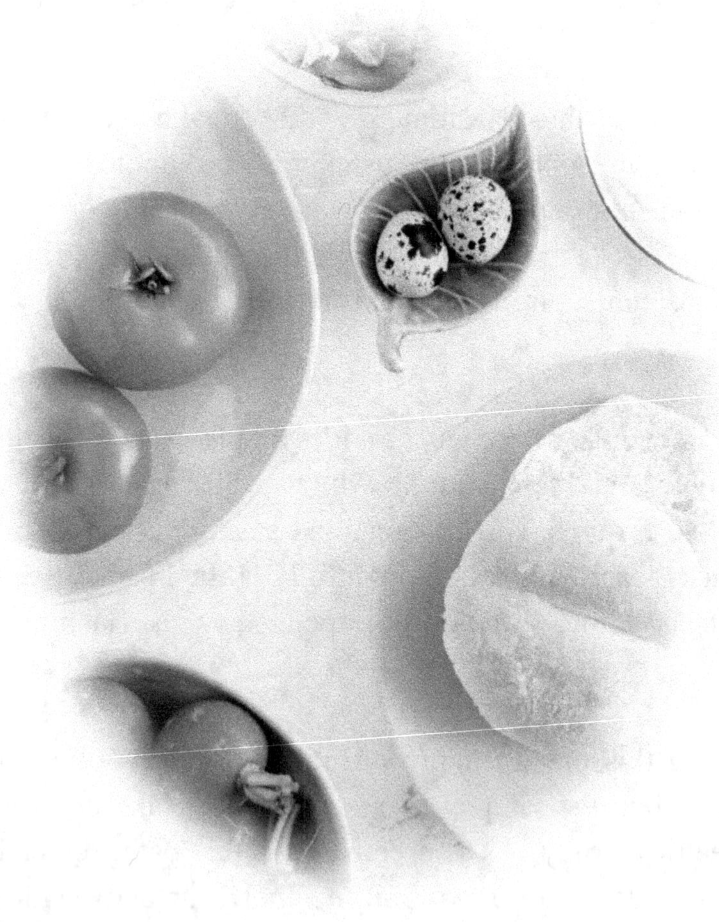

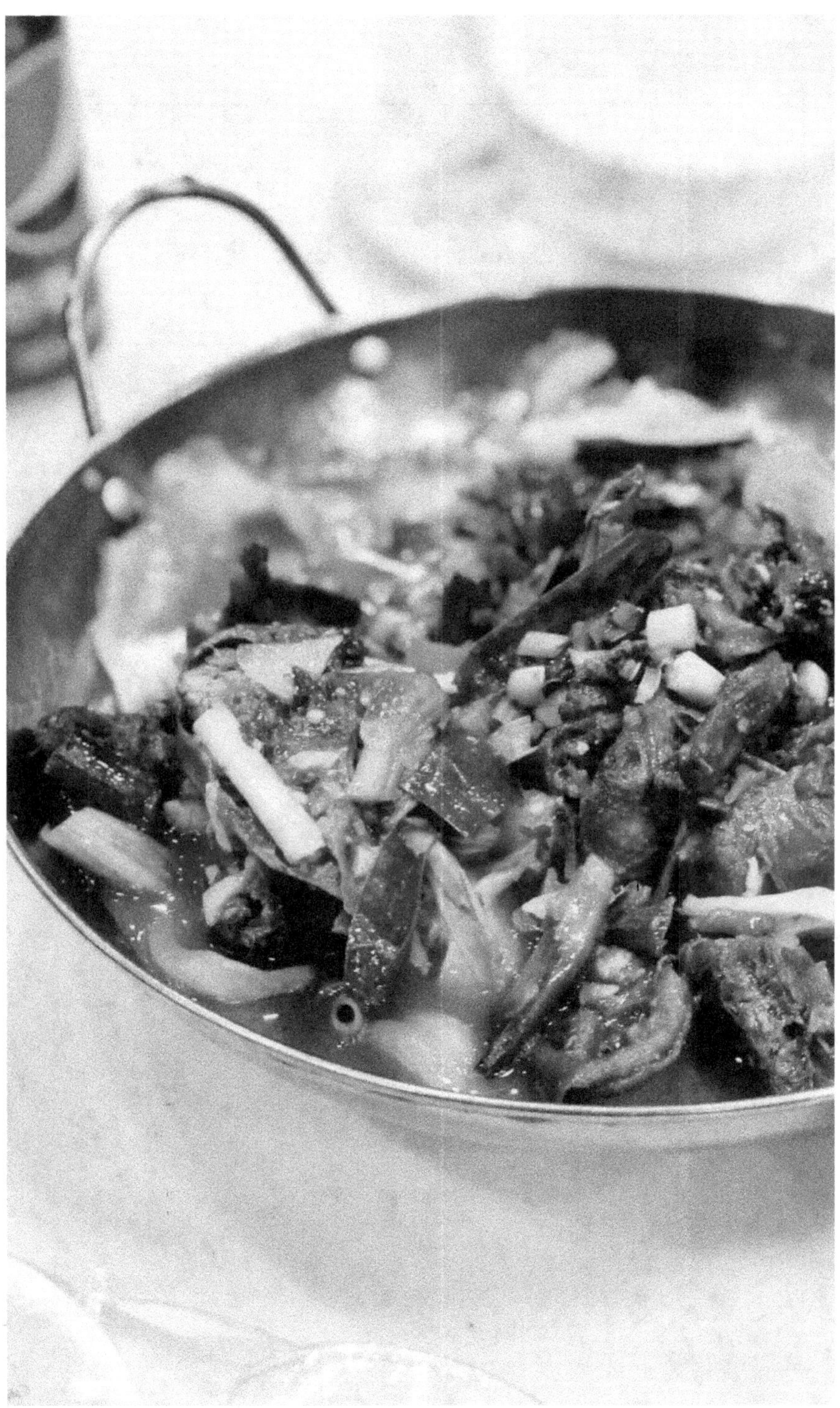

14-DAYS
Meal Plan

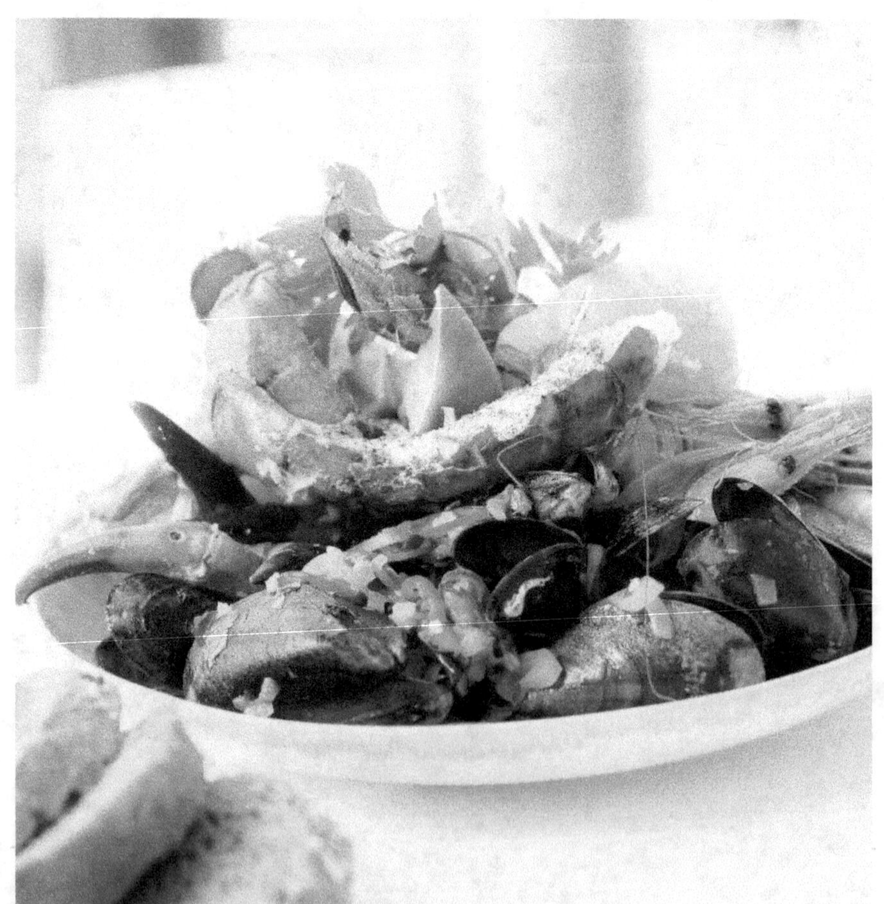

DAY	BREAK FAST	LUNCH	DINNER	SNACK
MONDAY	Quinoa-Stuffed Bell Peppers	Grilled Lemon Herb Shrimp Skewers	Lemon Garlic Roasted Chicken	Sliced cucumber with hummus
TUESDAY	Stuffed Sweet Potatoes with Black Beans and Avocado	Salmon and Avocado Salad with Citrus Dressing	Spicy Turkey Chili with Beans	Greek yogurt (dairy-free) with berries
WEDNESDAY	Mediterranean Stuffed Acorn Squash	Grilled Lemon Herb Salmon	Creamy Avocado Pasta with Grilled Chicken	Handful of mixed nuts
THURSDAY	Zucchini Noodles with Pesto and Cherry Tomatoes	Baked Lemon Garlic Tilapia	Stuffed Bell Peppers with Quinoa and Black Beans	Carrot sticks with almond butter
FRIDAY	Quinoa-Stuffed Bell Peppers	Lemon Garlic Roasted Chicken	Lemon Garlic Roasted Chicken	Sliced bell peppers with guacamole
SATURDAY	Stuffed Sweet Potatoes with Black Beans and Avocado	Grilled Lemon Herb Salmon	Spicy Turkey Meatballs with Tomato Sauce	Rice cakes with mashed avocado and tomato slices
SUNDAY	Mediterranean Stuffed Acorn Squash	Baked Lemon Garlic Tilapia	Creamy Avocado Pasta with Grilled Chicken	Greek yogurt (dairy-free) with berries

DAY	BREAK FAST	LUNCH	DINNER	SNACK
MONDAY	Zucchini Noodles with Pesto and Cherry Tomatoes	Grilled Lemon Herb Shrimp Skewers	Lemon Garlic Roasted Chicken	Sliced cucumber with hummus
TUESDAY	Quinoa-Stuffed Bell Peppers	Baked Lemon Garlic Tilapia	Coconut Curry Shrimp with Cauliflower Rice	Handful of mixed nuts
WEDNESDAY	Stuffed Sweet Potatoes with Black Beans and Avocado	Lemon Garlic Roasted Chicken	Spicy Turkey Meatballs with Tomato Sauce	Carrot sticks with almond butter
THURSDAY	Mediterranean Stuffed Acorn Squash	Grilled Lemon Herb Salmon	Creamy Avocado Pasta with Grilled Chicken	Sliced bell peppers with guacamole
FRIDAY	Zucchini Noodles with Pesto and Cherry Tomatoes	Grilled Lemon Herb Shrimp Skewers	Lemon Garlic Roasted Chicken	Rice cakes with mashed avocado and tomato slices
SATURDAY	Quinoa-Stuffed Bell Peppers	Baked Lemon Garlic Tilapia	Coconut Curry Shrimp with Cauliflower Rice	Greek yogurt (dairy-free) with berries
SUNDAY	Stuffed Sweet Potatoes with Black Beans and Avocado	Lemon Garlic Roasted Chicken	Spicy Turkey Meatballs with Tomato Sauce	Handful of mixed nuts

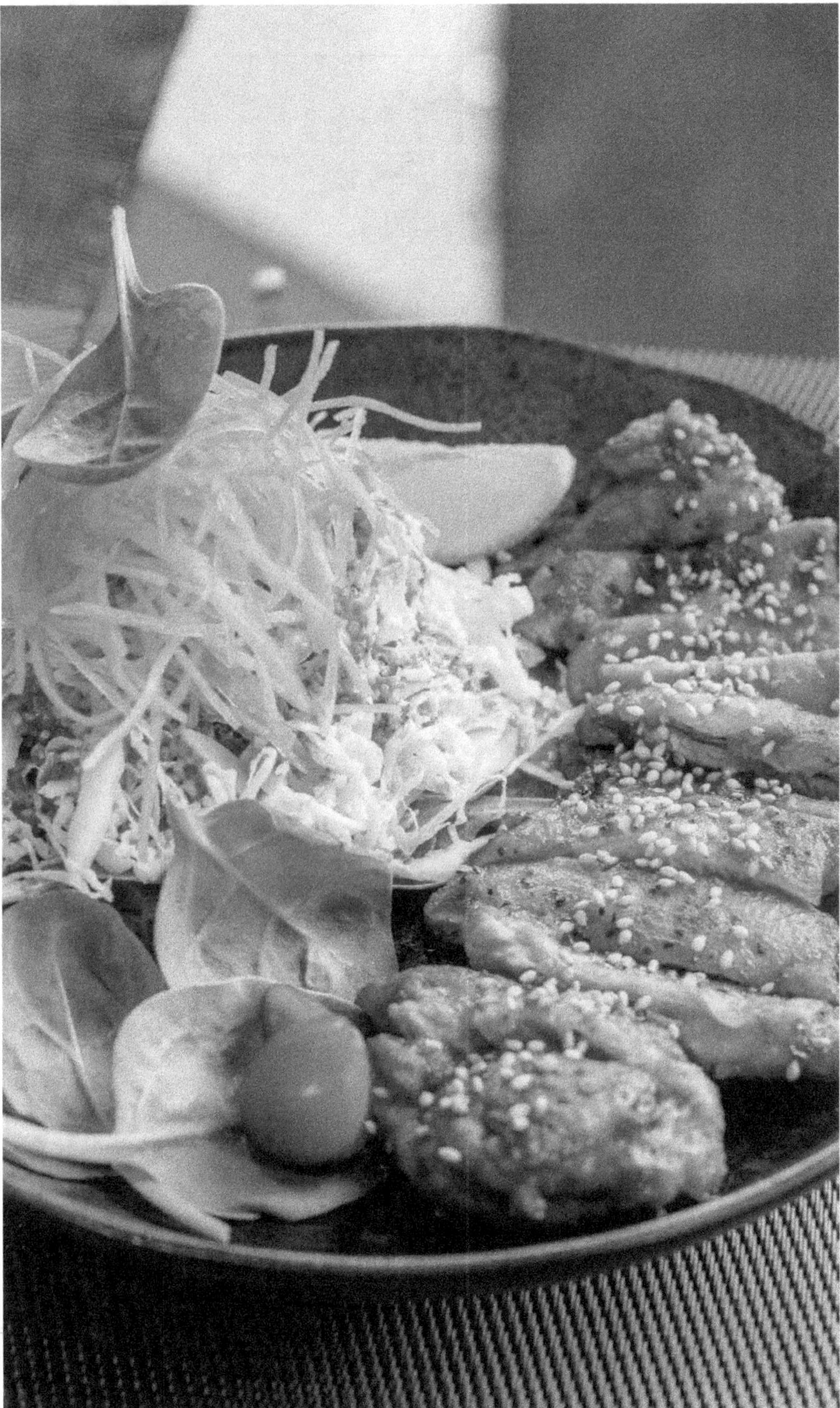

Weekly Meal *PLAN*

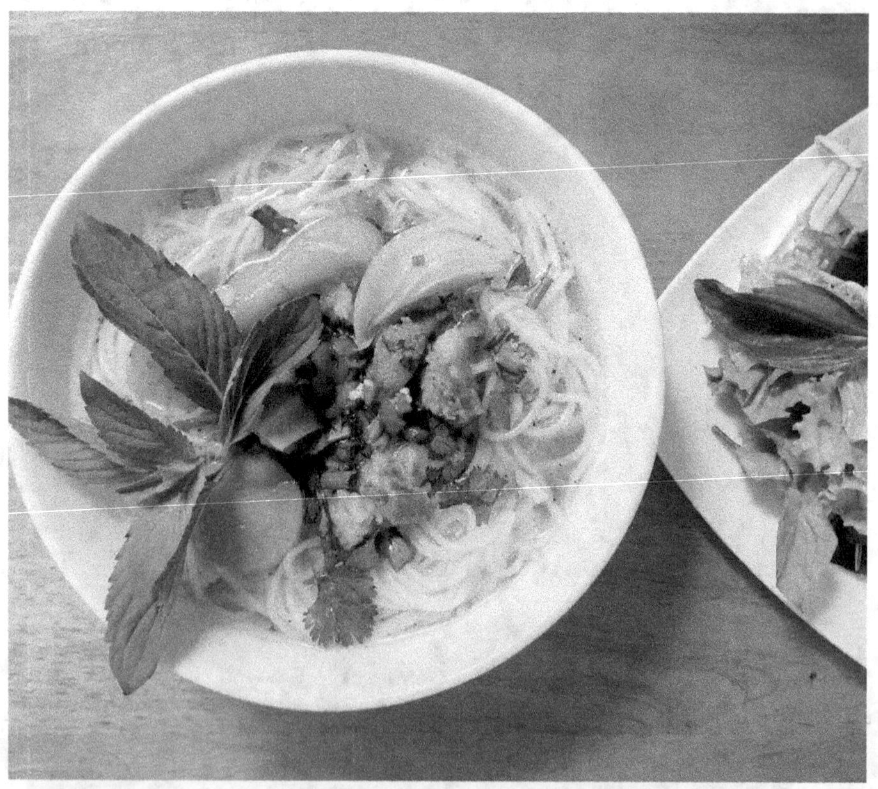

MEAL PLANNER

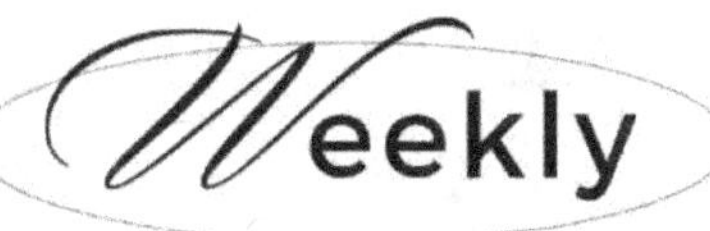

WEEK ____________________   MONTH ____________________

| MONDAY | SATURDAY |

| TUESDAY | SUNDAY |

| WEDNESDAY | **SHOPPING LIST** |

| THURSDAY |

| FRIDAY |

MEAL PLANNER

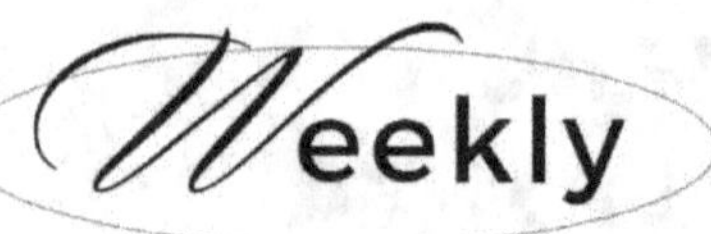

WEEK _______________________   MONTH _______________________

MONDAY

SATURDAY

TUESDAY

SUNDAY

WEDNESDAY

SHOPPING LIST

THURSDAY

FRIDAY

MEAL PLANNER

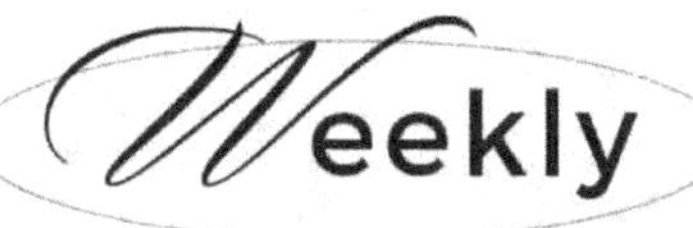

WEEK _______________

MONTH _______________

MONDAY

TUESDAY

WEDNESDAY

THURSDAY

FRIDAY

SATURDAY

SUNDAY

SHOPPING LIST

MEAL PLANNER

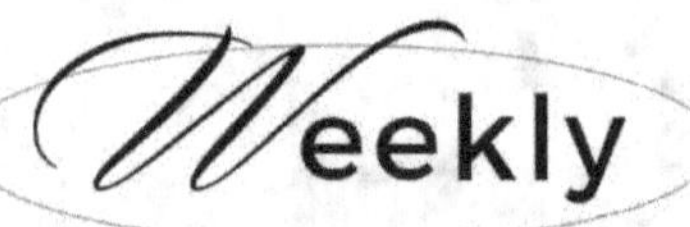

WEEK ___________________   MONTH ___________________

MONDAY

SATURDAY

TUESDAY

SUNDAY

WEDNESDAY

SHOPPING LIST

THURSDAY

FRIDAY

MEAL PLANNER

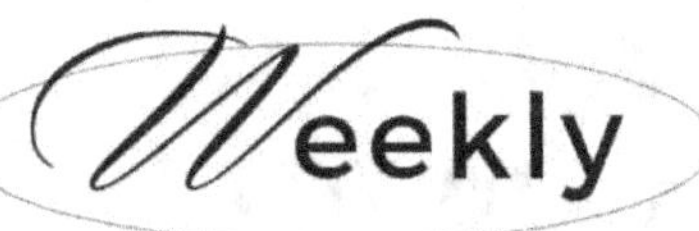

WEEK _______________   MONTH _______________

| MONDAY | SATURDAY |

| TUESDAY | SUNDAY |

| WEDNESDAY | **SHOPPING LIST** |

| THURSDAY | |

| FRIDAY | |

MEAL PLANNER

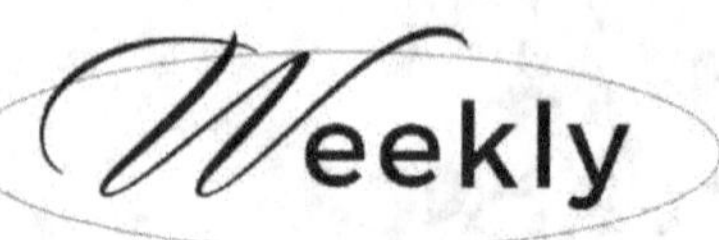

WEEK ___________________   MONTH ___________________

MONDAY

SATURDAY

TUESDAY

SUNDAY

WEDNESDAY

SHOPPING LIST

- ◯
- ◯
- ◯
- ◯
- ◯
- ◯
- ◯
- ◯
- ◯
- ◯
- ◯
- ◯
- ◯

THURSDAY

FRIDAY

MEAL PLANNER

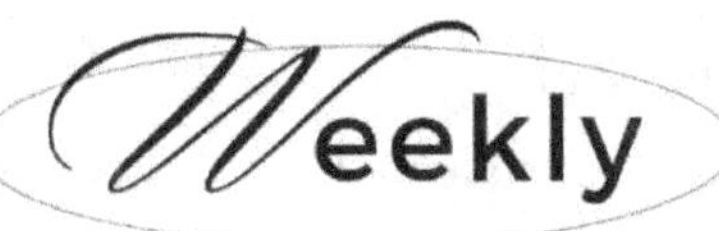

WEEK _______________________   MONTH _______________________

MONDAY

TUESDAY

WEDNESDAY

THURSDAY

FRIDAY

SATURDAY

SUNDAY

SHOPPING LIST

MEAL PLANNER

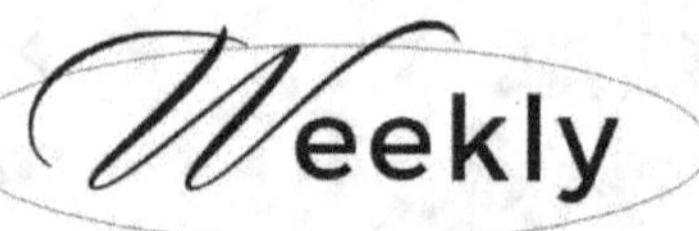

WEEK ___________________   MONTH ___________________

| MONDAY | SATURDAY |

| TUESDAY | SUNDAY |

WEDNESDAY

THURSDAY

FRIDAY

SHOPPING LIST

MEAL PLANNER

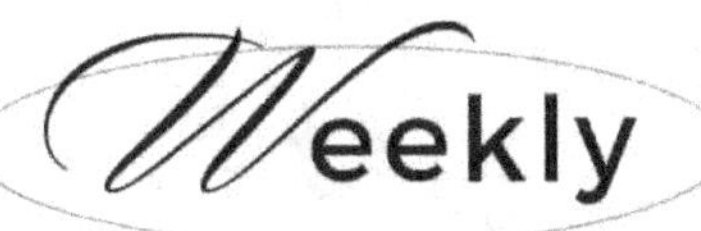

WEEK _______________   MONTH _______________

| MONDAY | SATURDAY |

| TUESDAY | SUNDAY |

| WEDNESDAY | SHOPPING LIST |

| THURSDAY | |

| FRIDAY | |

MEAL PLANNER

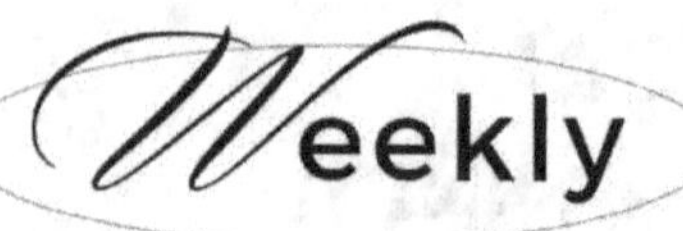

WEEK ________________________   MONTH ________________________

MONDAY

TUESDAY

WEDNESDAY

THURSDAY

FRIDAY

SATURDAY

SUNDAY

SHOPPING LIST

www.ingramcontent.com/pod-product-compliance
Lightning Source LLC
Chambersburg PA
CBHW071038250726

48653CB00005B/1880